SOMATIC EXERCISES FOR BEGINNERS

FUNDAMENTAL TECHNIQUES FOR WEIGHT LOSS, STRESS RELIEF, AND EMOTIONAL BALANCE

OLIVIA WELLNESS

UNDERSTANDING THE CONCEPT OF SOMATIC EXERCISES

Welcome to the world of somatic exercises, a realm where movement and mindfulness converge to create a harmonious experience for both the body and mind. At its core, the concept of somatic exercises revolves around the idea of internal physical perception and awareness. These practices are not just about moving the body; they are about connecting with and understanding it on a deeper level. Somatic exercises stem from the belief that our bodies hold not just physical strength and ability but also emotions and psychological states. By practicing these exercises, we learn to release tension, ease physical discomfort, and improve movement efficiency. More than that, we develop a profound connection with our inner selves, which can lead to a more balanced and fulfilling life: somatic exercises offer a unique approach to physical activity. Unlike traditional exercise routines that often focus on external goals such as muscle building or weight loss, somatic exercises encourage you to turn your attention inward. This shift in focus is not only beneficial for physical health but also promotes mental and emotional well-being. In this book, "Somatic Exercises for Beginners," you will embark on a journey of self-discovery through movement. You will learn how these exercises can help you become more in tune with your body, allowing for greater ease of movement and a better understanding of your physical self. As you progress through the book, you will find that somatic exercises are not just exercises; they are a form of self-care and a pathway to holistic wellness. The journey ahead is one of exploration and learning. As you delve into the practice of somatic exercises, you will uncover the subtle ways in which your body communicates and how you can respond to its needs. This introduction serves as the first step in understanding the foundational concepts of somatic exercises. It sets the stage for a transformative experience that goes beyond traditional exercise, offering a pathway to a more connected and mindful way of living in your body.

Let's begin this journey together with an open mind and a willingness to explore the depths of what your body can teach you.

The Benefits of Somatic Exercises for Beginners

Embarking on the journey of somatic exercises, especially as a beginner, opens the door to a myriad of benefits that extend beyond the physical realm. These exercises focused on the mind-body connection, offer a holistic approach to wellness that can profoundly impact various aspects of your life. One of the primary benefits of somatic exercises is the enhancement of body awareness. As you engage in these mindful movements, you begin to develop a deeper understanding of how your body operates. This heightened awareness leads to improved posture and movement efficiency as you become more attuned to the nuances of how your body feels and responds to different activities; Somatic exercises also offer an effective way to reduce stress and tension. The practice encourages you to focus on the present moment and the sensations within your body, which helps in calming the mind and reducing anxiety. This mindful approach to movement can be a powerful tool in managing everyday stress, leading to a more relaxed and balanced state of mind. Additionally, somatic exercises are known for their ability to alleviate physical discomfort and pain, particularly those stemming from habitual postures or repetitive strain. By learning to move your body in more natural and efficient ways, you can address underlying muscle tension and imbalances, often leading to a significant reduction in discomfort and an increase in overall physical comfort. For those new to exercise or returning after a break, somatic exercises provide a gentle and approachable way to begin. They focus on gentle movements that can be easily adapted to suit different fitness levels and physical conditions. This adaptability makes somatic exercises an inclusive practice, suitable for a wide range of individuals. Moreover, these exercises can improve flexibility and strength in a gentle, sustainable way. Unlike more intense workout regimens, somatic exercises encourage gradual progress, focusing on movements that naturally stretch and strengthen the body without the risk of injury. Lastly, somatic exercises can play a crucial role in emotional well-being. The practice of focusing inward and connecting with your body can lead to more excellent emotional balance and a sense of inner peace. It allows for a space where you can release pent-up emotions and find a sense of calmness in your daily life.

Somatic exercises offer beginners a comprehensive approach to wellness. They not only improve physical health and flexibility but also contribute significantly to mental and emotional well-being. As you begin your journey with these exercises, you'll likely find that their benefits extend well beyond the time spent practicing them, influencing various aspects of your daily life positively and holistically.

How to Approach Somatic Exercises as a Beginner

Approaching somatic exercises as a beginner can be both exciting and a little daunting. Still, with the right mindset and approach, it can become an enriching and transformative experience. Here are some key considerations to help you embark on this journey effectively:

1. Start with an Open Mind: As a beginner, it's crucial to approach somatic exercises with an open and curious mind. Let go of any preconceived notions about fitness and exercise. Be ready to explore a new way of connecting with your body.

2. Embrace the Basics: Begin with the fundamental principles of

somatic exercises. Focus on learning the basic movements and understanding how they feel in your body rather than trying to perfect them or achieve immediate results.

3. Listen to Your Body: One of the core aspects of somatic exercises is developing a deep listening to your body's signals. Pay attention to how each movement feels, and respect your body's limits. This practice is not about pushing through pain but rather about moving in ways that feel good and natural.

4. Prioritize Quality over Quantity: In somatic exercises, how you move is more important than how much or how often. Concentrate on the quality of each movement, ensuring you're performing them with mindfulness and care.

5. Regular Practice: Consistency is key. Try to incorporate somatic exercises into your routine, even if it's just for a few minutes each day. Regular practice will help you gradually build your skills and deepen your understanding of your body.

6. Utilize Resources: As you're learning, don't hesitate to use resources like books, videos, or even classes, if available. These can provide valuable guidance and ensure that you're on the right track.

7. Be Patient with Progress: Progress in somatic exercises can sometimes feel subtle. It's essential to be patient and recognize that even minor improvements in body awareness and movement efficiency are significant achievements.

8. Reflect on Your Journey: After each session, take a moment to reflect on your experience. How do you feel physically and mentally? What did you learn about your body? This reflection can deepen your practice and enhance the benefits.

9. Seek Guidance When Needed: If you need clarification on a movement or how to approach the exercises, feel free to seek guidance from a professional. A trained instructor can provide personalized advice and adjustments.

10. Enjoy the Process: Lastly, remember to enjoy the process of learning and exploring your body through somatic exercises. This journey is as much about the experience and the insights you gain along the way as it is about the physical benefits.

Approaching somatic exercises with these considerations in mind will set a strong foundation for your practice. As a beginner, each step you take in this journey is an opportunity to explore, learn, and grow in your understanding of your body and your overall well-being.

1

THE PHILOSOPHY OF SOMATIC EXERCISES

The journey into somatic exercises is rooted in a rich history and a profound philosophy that underscores the deep connection between the mind and the body. Understanding this history and evolution is essential for anyone embarking on the practice of somatic exercises, especially beginners. Somatic exercises emerged from a blend of Eastern and Western practices, intertwining ancient wisdom with modern scientific understanding of the human body. The word "somatic" is derived from the Greek word "soma," which means the living body in its wholeness. This concept dates back to ancient civilizations, where movement and the body's wisdom were integral to health and well-being. In the Western world, the foundation of somatic exercises can be traced back to the early 20th century. During this time, pioneers like F.M. Alexander (of the Alexander Technique), Moshe Feldenkrais (of the Feldenkrais Method), and Thomas Hanna (of Hanna Somatics) began exploring the relationship between movement, awareness, and the mind. They observed that by changing physical movement patterns, one could improve overall health, reduce pain, and increase the efficiency of movement. Throughout the 20th century, these practices evolved as more research and understanding emerged about the neurophysiology of the body. Somatic exercises began to incorporate principles from neuroscience, psychology, dance, and physical therapy. This multidisciplinary approach highlighted the importance of internal physical experience – how we feel our movements from within – as a pathway to healing and wellness.

Today, somatic exercises are recognized for their ability to foster self-awareness, enhance physical alignment, improve mobility, and reduce stress. They are used in various settings, including rehabilitation, fitness, stress management, and personal development. The practices have been adapted and expanded upon, giving rise to various schools and methods, each with its unique focus and techniques. At its core, the philosophy of somatic exercises is based on the idea that the mind and body are not separate entities but are intricately connected and interdependent. This holistic approach views movement not just as a physical activity but as a doorway to greater self-awareness and well-being. The practice encourages a mindful exploration of movements, fostering a dialogue between the body and the mind. The history and evolution of somatic practices reveal a continuous journey toward understanding the human body and its potential for healing, growth, and transformation; delving into this history offers not just context but also a deeper appreciation of the philosophy that underpins somatic exercises. It's a philosophy that advocates for a harmonious balance between the body and the mind, promoting a holistic approach to health and wellness that is as relevant today as it was in its inception.

As we explore the philosophy of bodily exercises, it becomes evident that this practice is anchored in a set of key principles. These principles form the backbone of somatic movements and offer a deeper understanding of their transformative potential. Firstly, the principle of mindfulness is central to somatic exercises. This involves a heightened awareness of one's physical sensations and movements. Unlike traditional exercises, where the focus might be on repetition or intensity, somatic exercises encourage a conscious, reflective approach. Practitioners are guided to pay close attention to how each movement feels, the subtle changes in muscle tension, and the rhythm of their breath. This mindful practice fosters a deeper connection between the body and the mind. Another fundamental principle is the concept of body awareness. Somatic exercises are designed to enhance one's understanding and perception of one's own body. This heightened awareness allows for a recognition of habitual patterns of movement and posture that may contribute to discomfort or inefficiency. By becoming more aware of these patterns, individuals can begin to alter them, leading to improved posture, reduced pain, and greater ease of movement. The principle of holistic movement is also key in somatic exercises. This approach views the body as an interconnected whole, where each part affects and is affected by the others. Somatic movements, therefore, focus on the body as a unit, moving away from isolated exercises. This holistic approach ensures that the exercises benefit the entire body, promoting overall balance and functional fitness. Relaxation and the release of tension are also central to somatic practices. Unlike exercise routines that emphasize exertion, somatic exercises often involve movements that encourage the muscles to relax and let go of chronic tension. This aspect is particularly beneficial for those dealing with stress-related physical issues, as it enables the body to release pent-up stress and rejuvenate. Lastly, the principle of adaptation and personalization makes somatic exercises accessible and effective for a wide range of individuals. Recognizing that each body is unique, somatic exercises can be adapted to fit the needs, abilities, and limitations of each person. This adaptable nature ensures that everyone, regardless of their physical condition or experience level, can benefit from the practice. These fundamental principles collectively contribute to the effectiveness and uniqueness of somatic exercises. They guide the practice toward not just physical fitness but also mental clarity, emotional balance, and overall well-being. For beginners, understanding these principles provides a solid foundation for their practice. It helps them reap the full benefits of somatic exercises.

The essence of somatic exercises lies in the profound understanding of the mind-body connection. This concept is both ancient and increasingly validated by modern science. This connection is not just a philosophical idea but a practical approach to wellness that somatic exercises beautifully illustrate and utilize. In somatic exercises, the mind and body are not viewed as separate entities but as parts of a unified whole. This holistic view recognizes that emotional, mental, and physical health are deeply intertwined. For instance, mental stress can manifest as physical tension, while physical discomfort can impact mental and emotional well-being. Somatic exercises aim to bridge this gap, using physical movement as a means to influence and improve mental and emotional states. Central to this approach is the concept of embodied cognition, which suggests that the body influences the mind just as the mind influences the body. In practice, this means that by changing how you move and hold your body, you can alter your mental and emotional state. Somatic exercises leverage this concept by encouraging movements that promote relaxation, awareness, and ease. These movements help to calm the mind, reduce stress, and foster a sense of emotional balance.

The practice of somatic exercises also involves a high degree of introspection and internal focus. Participants are encouraged to tune into their bodily sensations during movements – to notice the subtleties of muscle tension, the quality of their breathing, and the feelings that arise. This introspective process enhances body awareness and mindfulness, leading to a deeper understanding of the self. Moreover, somatic exercises often lead to the release of physical tension that has been held in the body, sometimes for years. This release can have a cathartic effect, not just physically but emotionally too. Many practitioners find that as their bodies let go of chronic tension, they also release the emotional burdens they have been carrying, leading to a feeling of lightness and emotional freedom. The mind-body connection in somatic exercises opens a pathway to holistic health. It offers a way to harmonize physical fitness with mental clarity and emotional resilience. This connection is the thread that runs through all somatic practices, making them not just exercises for the body, but nourishment for the mind and soul as well. Embracing this connection can lead to profound changes, not just in how you move but in how you feel, think, and engage with the world.

2

PREPARING FOR SOMATIC EXERCISES

In the journey through somatic exercises, especially for beginners, the importance of creating a conducive environment for practice cannot be overstated. This environment plays a crucial role in facilitating a deeper connection with the exercises, allowing you to immerse in the experience and reap maximum benefits fully.

Choosing the Right Space

The first step in creating a conducive environment is selecting an appropriate space for your practice. Ideally, this space should be quiet, comfortable, and free from distractions. It doesn't need to be large, but it should offer enough room for you to move freely. This could be a dedicated corner in your home, a peaceful spot in your garden, or any area that feels safe and calming. The key is to have a space where you can focus inward without external interruptions.

Setting the Ambiance

The ambiance of your practice space significantly influences your ability to relax and concentrate. Consider softening the lighting or using candles to create a tranquil atmosphere. Some practitioners find that gentle, soothing music or the sounds of nature can enhance their somatic experience. However, ensure that these elements are not distracting but rather supportive of your mindfulness and body awareness.

Gathering Your Tools

While somatic exercises don't require a lot of equipment, a few items can enhance your comfort and effectiveness. A yoga mat or a soft rug can provide cushioning and define your practice area. You should also have a blanket or a towel handy for specific exercises or relaxation at the end of your session. Comfortable clothing that allows for unrestricted movement is essential, as it helps you perform the exercises without constriction.

Mental Preparation

Creating a conducive environment also involves mental preparation. Before you begin your practice, take a few moments to transition from the busyness of your day to a state of calm focus. This might involve some deep breathing, a short meditation, or simply sitting quietly and setting an intention for your practice. This mental shift is as significant as the physical space in ensuring a beneficial somatic exercise session.

Consistency in Practice

Finally, try to practice in the same space consistently. Over time, this consistency will help condition your mind and body to enter a state of mindfulness and readiness for somatic exercises more quickly. Your practice space will become a personal sanctuary for growth, healing, and exploration.

Creating a conducive environment for somatic exercises is about more than just finding a physical space. It's about cultivating an atmosphere that supports mindfulness, introspection, and connection with your body. This environment becomes a crucial ally in your journey through somatic exercises, helping you achieve a deeper level of practice and understanding.

Embarking on the journey of somatic exercises, especially for beginners, requires little in the way of equipment and attire. Still, the right choices in these areas can significantly enhance the experience. The beauty of somatic exercises lies in their simplicity and the fact that they focus more on the internal experience rather than external accessories. However, having a few essentials can aid in ensuring comfort, safety, and the effectiveness of your practice. When it comes to attire, the key is to wear clothing that allows for unrestricted movement. This could be anything comfortable, breathable, and stretchable. The ideal attire would be similar to what one might wear for yoga or a light workout – leggings or shorts and a fitted top that stays in place as you move. The fit is important as overly loose clothing can sometimes get in the way of movement or obscure your view of your body, making it harder to maintain awareness of your posture and alignment. As for equipment, one of the most important items is a good quality exercise mat. A mat provides not just comfort but also safety, offering a non-slip surface that is essential for many somatic exercises. The thickness of the mat can vary based on personal preference and the type of floor you will be practicing on. If you're on a more complex surface, a thicker mat can provide more cushioning. Another helpful item, although optional, is a blanket. A blanket can be used for additional support and cushioning in various positions. It can also be helpful in maintaining warmth during relaxation or meditation exercises that conclude a somatic session.

It's also worth considering the space in which you'll be practicing. If you're in a room with a hard floor, you should have a softer area, like a rug or a carpeted section, where you can practice comfortably. Conversely, if you're on a very soft surface, you might want a firmer mat to provide better support. In addition to these physical preparations, there's also an aspect of mental preparation that involves gearing up for the practice. This doesn't require any physical equipment but involves preparing your mind for a session of introspective and mindful movement. Taking a few moments before starting to clear your mind, setting intentions for your practice, or simply tuning into your breath can be incredibly beneficial. In essence, while somatic exercises don't require a lot of equipment, having the proper attire and a few essential items can help create a more comfortable and focused practice environment. These tools are there to support your journey into somatic exercises, making the experience as enriching and beneficial as possible.

Understanding your body's signals and boundaries is a fundamental aspect of beginning somatic exercises. This practice is not just about executing movements; it's about developing a deep and intuitive connection with your body. It requires listening closely to what your body is telling you and respecting its limits, which is a vital skill for beginners to cultivate.

In somatic exercises, every movement and pose is an opportunity to engage in a dialogue with your body. It's essential to pay attention to how different movements feel. Do they bring a sense of ease and release, or do they lead to discomfort or strain? Learning to differentiate between a beneficial stretch and a harmful strain is crucial. A good stretch can feel like a gentle pull, helping to release tension and increase flexibility. In contrast, a painful strain is a clear signal from your body that you are pushing too far and need to ease back. Breathing patterns are also insightful indicators. Smooth, steady breathing suggests that you are working within your comfort zone. On the other hand, if your breath becomes rapid and shallow, or if you find yourself holding your breath, it could be a sign that you're exerting beyond your current capabilities. Fatigue is another important signal. While some level of fatigue is expected in any physical practice, it's essential to distinguish between the healthy tiredness that comes from a satisfying workout and the exhaustion that results from overexertion. If you feel drained rather than energized after a session, it might be time to scale back and allow more time for rest and recovery. Moreover, being aware of your emotional responses during and after exercises can provide valuable insights. Somatic exercises often release stored emotions, and it's not uncommon to experience a range of feelings during practice. Acknowledging and accepting these emotions as part of the process is an integral part of understanding your body's language. Give your body time to adjust to new movements and routines. It's better to err on the side of caution and gradually increase intensity than to push too hard and risk injury or burnout. Understanding and respecting your body's signals and boundaries are key to a safe and effective somatic exercise practice. By cultivating awareness and listening to your body, you ensure that your practice supports and enhances your well-being, paving the way for a rewarding and sustainable journey into somatic exercises.

3

FUNDAMENTAL TECHNIQUES AND CONCEPTS

As we delve into this Chapter of "Somatic Exercises for Beginners," we focus on the foundational elements of the practice, particularly the basic postures and their significance. These postures are the building blocks of somatic exercises, serving as the starting point from which you can explore and deepen your practice. The significance of these basic postures lies in their ability to establish a strong foundation for body awareness and movement efficiency. Each posture is designed not just to engage certain muscle groups but to enhance your overall body awareness. This awareness is crucial in learning how to move your body in ways that are both efficient and harmonious. One of the key aspects of these postures is their focus on alignment and balance. Proper alignment ensures that you are working your body symmetrically and reduces the risk of injury. It also ensures that you are engaging the correct muscles for each movement. This focus on alignment is not about achieving perfection in each posture but about understanding how slight adjustments in your position can significantly impact how the exercise feels and its effectiveness. The basic postures also serve as a tool for mindfulness. As you hold each posture, you are encouraged to pay close attention to your breathing, the sensations in your muscles, and the feelings that arise during the practice. This mindfulness aspect is what transforms these exercises from mere physical movements into a holistic practice that nurtures both the body and mind. Moreover, these postures are significant for their adaptability. They can be modified to suit various fitness levels and physical abilities, making somatic exercises inclusive and accessible to a wide range of people. Whether you are a complete beginner or someone with physical limitations, these postures can be adjusted to meet you where you are in your fitness journey.

Incorporating these basic postures into your routine is also a way to develop consistency in your practice. As you become familiar with these foundational elements, you'll find it easier to establish a routine, which is key to reaping the long-term benefits of somatic exercises. The basic postures in somatic exercises are much more than just physical positions. They are a means to connect with your body, enhance your awareness, and establish a solid foundation for your practice. As you learn and practice these postures, you embark on a journey of discovery, learning not just about the exercises themselves but also about your body and how it moves and feels. This chapter aims to guide you through that journey, helping you build the necessary skills and understanding to progress in your somatic exercise practice.

Breathing techniques hold a place of paramount importance in somatic exercises, especially for beginners. In this practice, how you breathe is not just a matter of drawing air in and out of your lungs; it's a vital component of how you connect with your body and mind. The way you breathe during somatic exercises can significantly influence the effectiveness of your movements and your overall experience. In somatic exercises, breath is often used as a tool to enhance awareness and deepen relaxation. Unlike some forms of exercise where breathing might be more automatic or secondary, here, it is brought to the forefront. You are encouraged to observe your breath, noticing the rhythm, depth, and patterns of your breathing. This observation is the first step in learning to use your breath intentionally in your practice. One common technique in somatic exercises is diaphragmatic breathing or belly breathing. This involves breathing deeply into your diaphragm rather than shallowly into your chest. As you inhale, your belly expands, and as you exhale, it contracts. This type of breathing is known to trigger relaxation responses in the body, helping to reduce stress and tension. Another aspect of breathing in somatic exercises is coordinating breath with movement. In many exercises, you'll find that inhaling accompanies one phase of a movement (often the expansion or opening phase). In contrast, exhaling accompanies another (often the contraction or closing phase). This coordination helps to create a harmonious flow of movement, enhancing the physical benefits of the exercise and bringing a sense of calm and focus to your practice. Breath can also be used as a tool to release tension. In some exercises, you may be guided to focus your breath on areas of tightness or discomfort in your body. Directing your breath to these areas helps facilitate a sense of release and ease: mastering these breathing techniques can take time and practice. It's essential to be patient and not force your breath. With regular practice, breathing in somatic exercises becomes more intuitive and can significantly enhance your experience of the movements. Breathing techniques in somatic exercises are about more than just supplying oxygen to your muscles; they are about creating a deeper connection between your body and mind. By learning to breathe effectively in your practice, you unlock a more significant potential for relaxation, awareness, and movement efficiency. This chapter aims to guide you through the various breathing techniques used in somatic exercises, helping you integrate them into your practice for a more holistic and enriching experience.

Developing body awareness and mindfulness is a cornerstone of somatic exercises, particularly for beginners. This practice is much more than a series of physical movements; it's a journey into deeper self-awareness and presence. At its heart, somatic exercises are about cultivating an intimate understanding of your own body and using that knowledge to move in more harmonious and healthful ways. Body awareness in the context of somatic exercises involves a heightened sense of how your body feels and moves in space. It's about tuning into the subtle sensations within your body - noticing how muscles engage and release, how joints move, and even how your weight shifts during various movements. This kind of awareness allows you to recognize patterns in your body, such as areas of tension or imbalance, and address them through your practice. It begins with simple observations - how does your breath feel as you inhale and exhale? How do your feet feel against the floor? As you progress, these observations become more nuanced, helping you understand your body's unique language and signals. Mindfulness, closely tied to body awareness, is about being fully present in the moment. In somatic exercises, mindfulness means paying close attention to each movement, each breath, and each sensation without judgment or distraction. This present-moment awareness enhances the connection between the mind and the body, allowing for a deeper engagement with the exercises. The practice of mindfulness in somatic exercises extends beyond physical movement. It includes being mindful of your thoughts and emotions as you practice. By acknowledging and accepting your thoughts and feelings without getting caught up in them, you can achieve a state of mental clarity and calm that complements the physical aspects of the exercises. The integration of body awareness and mindfulness might initially seem challenging. However, with regular practice, it becomes more accessible. It's a skill that grows over time, not only enriching your practice of somatic exercises but also spilling over into other areas of your life. Increased body awareness and mindfulness can lead to better posture, reduced stress, and an overall sense of well-being. Developing body awareness and mindfulness is about creating a deeper connection with yourself. It's about moving beyond mere physical fitness to a place where you are in tune with the subtle cues of your body and mind. This chapter aims to guide you through the process of cultivating these essential skills, laying the foundation for a fulfilling and effective practice of somatic exercises.

PRACTICAL SECTION

As you embark on the practical exercise section of this book, I'm excited to share with you the very same routines and poses that I offer to my private clients. These exercises have been carefully selected and structured to ensure that you can perform them independently and effectively, just by reading the descriptions. My aim is to provide you with clear, easy-to-understand instructions that empower you to carry out each movement with confidence and autonomy. Each pose and routine described in this book is crafted to be self-explanatory, eliminating the need for visual aids. The detailed descriptions are designed to guide you through each exercise, helping you visualize and execute the movements accurately. This approach fosters a deeper understanding and connection with your body, enhancing the effectiveness of each exercise.

While I strive to make each instruction as clear as possible, I understand that sometimes seeing a movement in action can provide additional clarity. If you find yourself needing a visual reference for any of the exercises, a simple search on a video platform like YouTube, using the name of the pose, can offer you supplementary guidance. This way, you can ensure you're performing each movement correctly and safely.

I have arranged a unique and user-friendly layout to enhance your learning and practice experience. Each left-hand page details a specific exercise, complete with its practical explanation. This approach is designed to guide you step-by-step through the execution of each movement, ensuring you can perform the exercise correctly and effectively.

On the right-hand page corresponding to each exercise, you'll find valuable tips and notes. These insights are aimed at enriching your understanding of the exercise, providing additional context, and offering guidance to refine your technique.

This dual-page layout has been thoughtfully designed to provide a comprehensive learning experience. It ensures that you have all the necessary information at your fingertips, facilitating a deeper engagement with each exercis. These additional insights will help you tailor the exercises to your individual needs and goals.

Remember, the journey to wellness is personal and ever-evolving. These exercises, along with the accompanying tips and notes, are here to support you on your path to improved health and well-being.

Levels of experience and fitness (you can combine them in the diary you'll find)

- **Warm-Up and Stretching**

These exercises are designed to prepare your body for the workout ahead. They include both dynamic and static stretching routines, perfect for getting your muscles ready and preventing injuries.

- **Basic Exercises**

Ideal for beginners or those looking to focus on body awareness and fluid movement, these exercises form the foundation of a good fitness routine.

- **Intermediate Exercises**

As you progress, these exercises will help you step up in terms of intensity and complexity, offering a balanced challenge for your developing skills.

Remember, this journey is about your personal growth and well-being. Each exercise is a step towards a healthier, more balanced you. Whether you're a beginner or an experienced fitness enthusiast, there's something in here for everyone.

WARM-UP EXERCISES TO PREPARE THE BODY

Jogging on the Spot

How to Perform Jogging on the Spot

1. Starting Position: Stand upright with your feet hip-width apart. Keep your back straight, shoulders relaxed, and look forward.
2. Arm Movement: Bend your arms at the elbows. As you jog, swing your arms back and forth in rhythm with your legs. Keep your hands relaxed.
3. Leg Movement: Begin to lift your feet off the ground in a light jogging motion. Your knees should lift slightly with each step.
4. Pace: Start with a slow pace to gradually warm up your body. As you feel more comfortable, you can increase the speed to raise your heart rate further.
5. Breathing: Maintain steady, even breaths. Inhale and exhale rhythmically to ensure a steady supply of oxygen during the exercise.
6. Duration: Continue jogging on the spot for about 3-5 minutes, depending on your fitness level.

Jogging on the Spot

Tips

- Keep your movements light and bouncy. Avoid heavy stomping to reduce impact on your joints.
- Focus on engaging your core muscles to maintain balance and stability.
- Keep your gaze forward and your head up to maintain a neutral neck position.

Note

Jogging on the spot is an excellent warm-up exercise as it gently increases your heart rate and warms up your muscles, preparing your body for more intensive workouts.

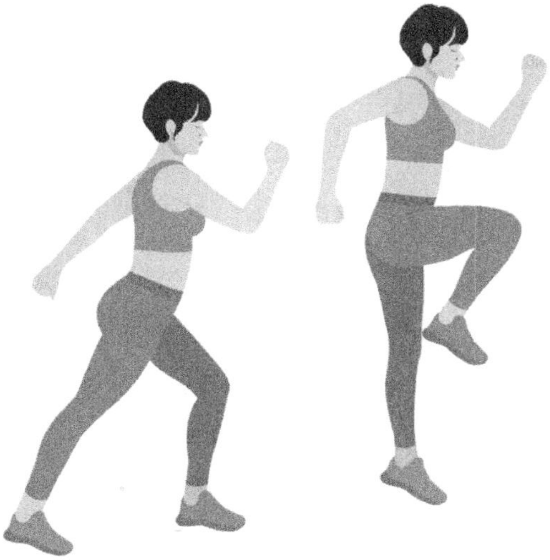

If you find yourself needing a visual reference for any of the exercises, a simple search on a video platform like YouTube, using the name of the pose, can offer you supplementary guidance. This way, you can ensure you're performing each movement correctly and safely.

Hip Circles

How to Perform Hip Circles

1. Starting Position: Stand with your feet shoulder-width apart. Keep your knees slightly bent for stability.
2. Hand Position: Place your hands on your hips or rest them on your waist.
3. The Movement: Gently push your hips forward, then to the side, backward, and to the other side, creating a circular motion. Imagine drawing a circle with your hips.
4. Range of Motion: Start with smaller circles, and as your hips begin to loosen, gradually increase the size of the circles.
5. Direction: After completing several circles in one direction, switch and rotate your hips in the opposite direction.
6. Rhythm and Breathing: Maintain a slow and controlled pace, coordinating your breath with the movement. Inhale as you move your hips forward and exhale as you move them backward.
7. Duration: Continue performing hip circles for about 1-2 minutes, or until you feel your hip area is adequately warmed up.

Hip Circles

Tips

- Keep your upper body as still as possible, focusing the movement in the hips.
- Avoid rushing the circles. The effectiveness of this exercise lies in its slow, deliberate motion.
- Pay attention to any tightness or restrictions in your hip movement and work within your comfortable range of motion.

Note

Hip circles are excellent for enhancing hip mobility, which is essential for overall lower body flexibility and function.

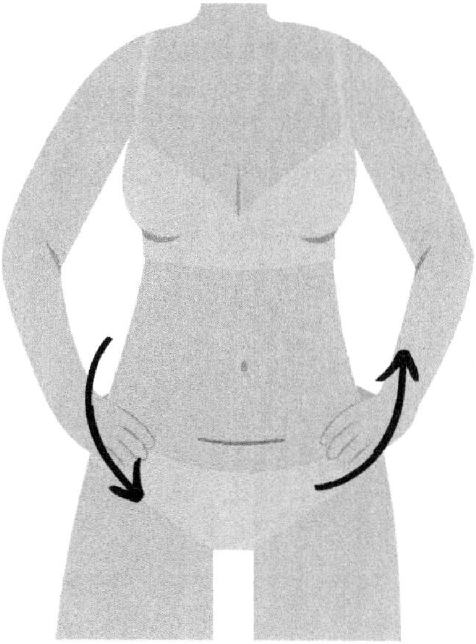

If you find yourself needing a visual reference for any of the exercises, a simple search on a video platform like YouTube, using the name of the pose, can offer you supplementary guidance. This way, you can ensure you're performing each movement correctly and safely.

Arm Swings

How to Perform Arm Swings

1. Starting Position: Stand with your feet shoulder-width apart. Keep your knees slightly bent and your back straight.
2. Arm Position: Extend your arms out to the sides at shoulder height.
3. The Movement: Begin to swing your arms gently in front of your body and then behind, in a steady and controlled motion. The arms should cross in front of your chest when swinging forward.
4. Range of Motion: Gradually increase the range of motion as your muscles warm up. Ensure that the movement is coming from your shoulders.
5. Rhythm and Breathing: Maintain a rhythmic pace and coordinate your breath with the movement – inhale as your arms swing back and exhale as they swing forward.
6. Duration: Continue the arm swings for about 30-60 seconds, or until you feel your shoulders and chest have warmed up.

Arm Swings

Tips

- Keep your movements fluid and avoid jerky motions to prevent strain.
- Focus on relaxing your shoulders as you swing your arms. Avoid tensing up your neck or upper back.
- As you progress, you can increase the speed of your swings slightly, but always prioritize control and range of motion over speed.

Note

Arm swings are an effective way to warm up the shoulders and chest, preparing them for more strenuous activities.

This is another method to practice this exercise

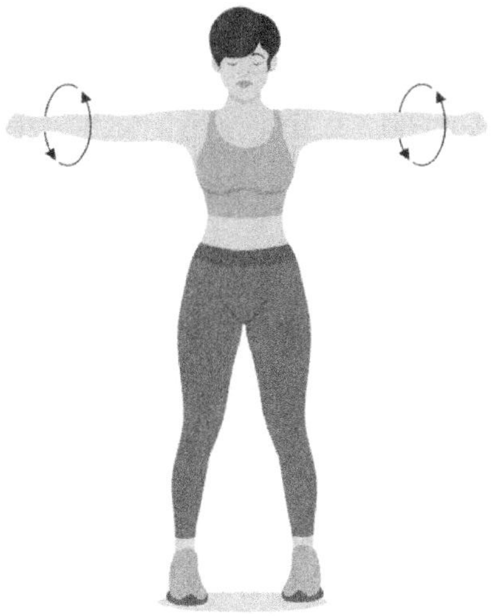

If you find yourself needing a visual reference for any of the exercises, a simple search on a video platform like YouTube, using the name of the pose, can offer you supplementary guidance. This way, you can ensure you're performing each movement correctly and safely.

Spinal Twists

How to Perform Spinal Twists

1. Starting Position: Sit on the floor with your legs extended in front of you. Keep your back straight and your shoulders relaxed.
2. Leg Position: Bend your right knee and place your right foot on the outside of your left knee. Keep your left leg straight or you can bend it with your left foot near your right buttock, if comfortable.
3. Twist Movement: Turn your upper body to the right. Place your left elbow on the outside of your right knee and your right hand on the floor behind you for support.
4. Gaze and Upper Body: As you twist, turn your head to look over your right shoulder if it's comfortable for your neck. Ensure that the twist is initiated from your lower back, moving up to the upper back, and then the neck.
5. Breathing: Inhale deeply as you sit up tall, and exhale as you deepen the twist. Keep your breathing steady and deep.
6. Hold and Switch Sides: Hold the twist for about 20-30 seconds, then release and repeat on the other side.

Spinal Twists

Tips

- It's important to keep your spine straight and elongated during the twist. Avoid slouching or rounding your back.
- Move into the twist gently and slowly. Do not force your body into a deeper twist than is comfortable.
- Focus on the sensation of the twist rather than how far you can turn. The aim is to increase spinal mobility, not to push into discomfort.
- If you experience any pain, especially in the lower back or neck, ease off the twist and consult with a healthcare professional if necessary.

Note

Spinal twists are excellent for increasing spinal mobility, improving digestion, and relieving tension in the back. They help to stretch the back muscles and spine, promoting flexibility and relaxation.

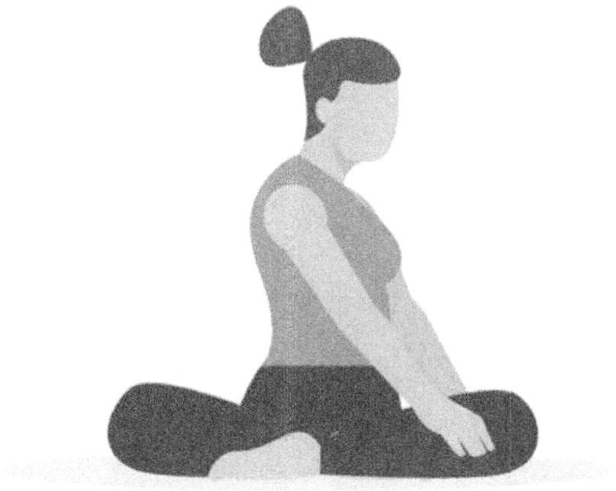

If you find yourself needing a visual reference for any of the exercises, a simple search on a video platform like YouTube, using the name of the pose, can offer you supplementary guidance. This way, you can ensure you're performing each movement correctly and safely.

Knee Lifts

How to Perform Knee Lifts

1. Starting Position: Stand tall with your feet hip-width apart. Keep your back straight, and your arms at your sides or place your hands on your hips for balance.
2. The Movement: Slowly lift one knee towards your chest while keeping the other leg straight and stable. Raise the knee as high as comfortably possible without straining.
3. Balance: Focus on maintaining your balance. If needed, hold onto a chair or wall for support.
4. Alternate Legs: Lower the lifted knee back to the starting position and then lift the other knee. Alternate between legs with a smooth and controlled motion.
5. Breathing: Inhale as you lift your knee and exhale as you lower it back down.
6. Duration: Perform this exercise for about 1-2 minutes, alternating knees.

Knee Lifts

Tips

- Keep your movements controlled. Avoid jerky or rushed motions to prevent any strain on your joints.
- Engage your core muscles throughout the exercise to help with balance and stability.
- Keep your lifted foot flexed to engage the muscles in your leg more effectively.
- As you progress, try to lift your knee higher to increase the range of motion and intensity of the exercise.

Note

Knee lifts are a great way to activate your leg muscles and glutes, and they also help improve balance and coordination.

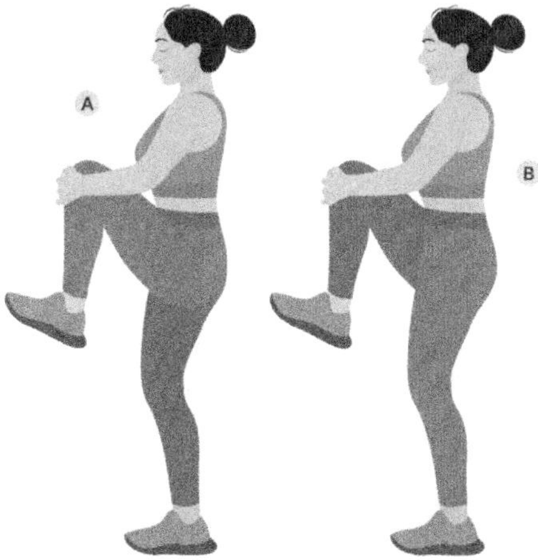

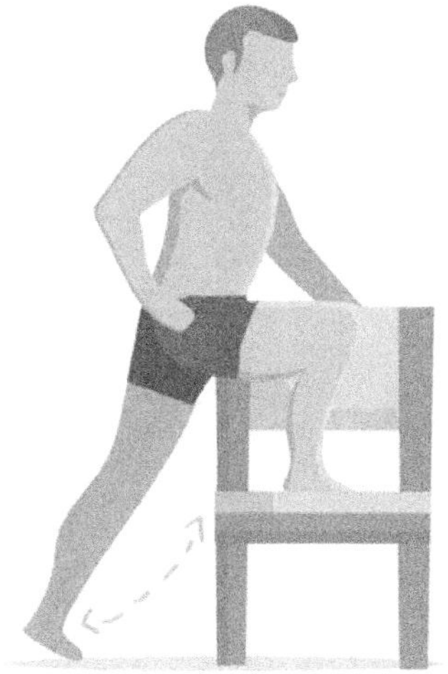

If you find yourself needing a visual reference for any of the exercises, a simple search on a video platform like YouTube, using the name of the pose, can offer you supplementary guidance. This way, you can ensure you're performing each movement correctly and safely.

DYNAMIC AND STATIC STRETCHING

Arm and Shoulder Stretch

How to Perform Arm and Shoulder Stretch

1. Starting Position: Stand with your feet shoulder-width apart. Keep your knees slightly bent and your body relaxed.
2. Arm Swings: Extend your arms out to your sides at shoulder height. Swing them slowly in front of your chest and then open them back out wide. Continue this movement in a controlled manner for about 30 seconds.
3. Shoulder Circles: Next, perform shoulder circles. Lift your shoulders up towards your ears, then roll them backward, down, and then forward in a circular motion. Do this for about 20 seconds, then reverse the direction for another 20 seconds.
4. Cross-Body Arm Stretch: Extend one arm straight across your chest. Use your other hand to gently pull the extended arm closer to your chest, stretching the shoulder. Hold for about 15 seconds, then switch arms.
5. Tricep Stretch: Lift one arm overhead, then bend your elbow so that your hand reaches towards the opposite shoulder blade. Use your other hand to gently press on the bent elbow for a deeper stretch. Hold for 15 seconds, then switch arms.
6. Rhythm and Breathing: Keep your movements smooth and coordinated with your breathing. Inhale during the initial phase of the stretch and exhale as you deepen the stretch.

Arm and Shoulder Stretch

Tips

- Ensure that your movements are fluid and controlled. Avoid jerking or bouncing, as this can cause muscle strain.
- For the cross-body and tricep stretches, be careful not to pull or push too hard. The stretch should feel comfortable and not painful.
- Keep your neck relaxed and your posture upright during the stretches. Avoid slumping or leaning to one side.
- If you feel any pain, especially in the shoulder joints, stop immediately and consult a healthcare professional.

Note

Arm and shoulder stretches are essential for maintaining flexibility and range of motion in the upper body. They are particularly beneficial for individuals who spend a lot of time at a desk or in front of a computer, as they help relieve tension and prevent stiffness in the arms, shoulders, and upper back. These dynamic stretches warm up the muscles, making them an excellent preparation for upper-body intensive activities.

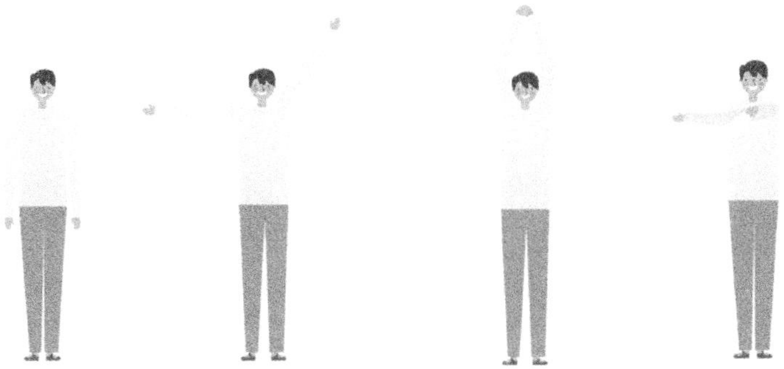

If you find yourself needing a visual reference for any of the exercises, a simple search on a video platform like YouTube, using the name of the pose, can offer you supplementary guidance. This way, you can ensure you're performing each movement correctly and safely.

Standing Toe Touches

How to Perform Standing Toe Touches

1. Starting Position: Stand with your feet hip-width apart. Keep your knees slightly bent to avoid strain on your lower back.
2. The Movement: Inhale and slowly extend your arms above your head. As you exhale, hinge at your hips and bend forward, reaching towards your toes. Keep your back straight as you lower down.
3. Touch and Return: Try to touch your toes, but if you can't reach them, go as far as comfortable, whether that's your shins or knees. Hold the position for a few seconds.
4. Rising Up: Inhale as you slowly roll back up to the standing position, vertebra by vertebra, keeping your back straight. Your head should come up last.
5. Repetition: Repeat this stretch 5-10 times, each time trying to stretch a little further, but always within your comfort zone.

Standing Toe Touches

Tips

- Focus on keeping the movement fluid and controlled. Avoid any jerky motions which can lead to muscle strain.
- It's important to keep the knees slightly bent, especially if you have tight hamstrings or lower back issues.
- This stretch targets the hamstrings and lower back, so you should feel a gentle pull in these areas, but no pain.
- Ensure that the bend is coming from your hips, not your waist, to maximize the stretch in the back of your legs.
- Breathe deeply throughout the stretch, as this will help deepen the stretch and relax your muscles.

Note

Standing toe touches are an excellent dynamic stretch for the back of the legs and the lower back. They help to improve flexibility in the hamstrings and can alleviate tension in the lower back, which is especially beneficial for those who sit for prolonged periods. This exercise also promotes blood flow to the upper body, making it a great choice for a warm-up or cool-down routine.

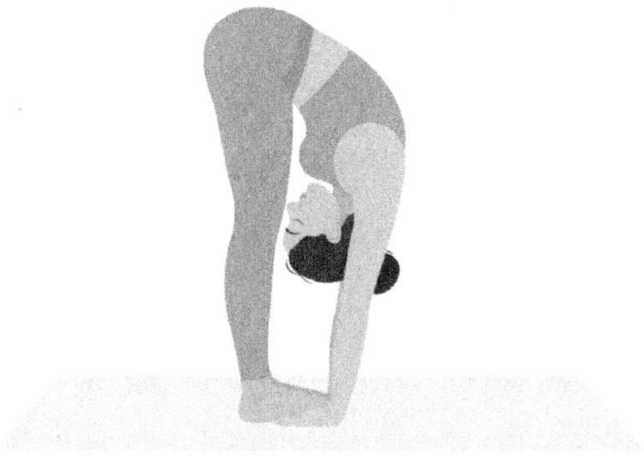

If you find yourself needing a visual reference for any of the exercises, a simple search on a video platform like YouTube, using the name of the pose, can offer you supplementary guidance. This way, you can ensure you're performing each movement correctly and safely.

Dynamic Leg Stretches

How to Perform Dynamic Leg Stretches

1. Starting Position: Stand upright with your feet hip-width apart. Keep your arms at your sides or place your hands on your hips for balance.
2. Forward Leg Swings: Begin with forward leg swings. Swing one leg forward and backward, gently increasing the range of motion. Keep your leg straight as you swing it, and avoid arching your back. Do this for about 30 seconds, then switch legs.
3. Side Leg Swings: Next, move to side leg swings. Stand sideways near a wall or a stable object for support. Swing your outside leg across the front of your body and then out to the side, again keeping the leg straight. Continue for about 30 seconds before switching to the other leg.
4. Lunging Stretch: Perform dynamic lunging stretches. Step forward into a lunge and lower your hips until your front thigh is parallel to the floor. Ensure your front knee doesn't go past your toes. Push back to the starting position and alternate legs. Continue for about 1 minute.
5. Rhythm and Breathing: Maintain a rhythmic pace and coordinate your breath with your movements. Inhale as you prepare for the stretch, and exhale as you execute the stretch.

Dynamic Leg Stretches

Tips

- Dynamic leg stretches should be performed in a controlled manner. Avoid jerky or overly forceful movements that could strain your muscles.
- Focus on warming up the muscles rather than stretching them to their limits. The goal is to prepare your muscles for more intense activity.
- As you progress, you can increase the speed and range of motion, but always listen to your body and stay within a comfortable range.
- Keep your core engaged during these stretches to support your back and improve balance.

Note

Dynamic leg stretches are ideal for warming up the leg muscles in motion, preparing them for a workout or physical activity. They help improve circulation, increase muscle temperature, and enhance flexibility, reducing the risk of injury during more strenuous exercises.

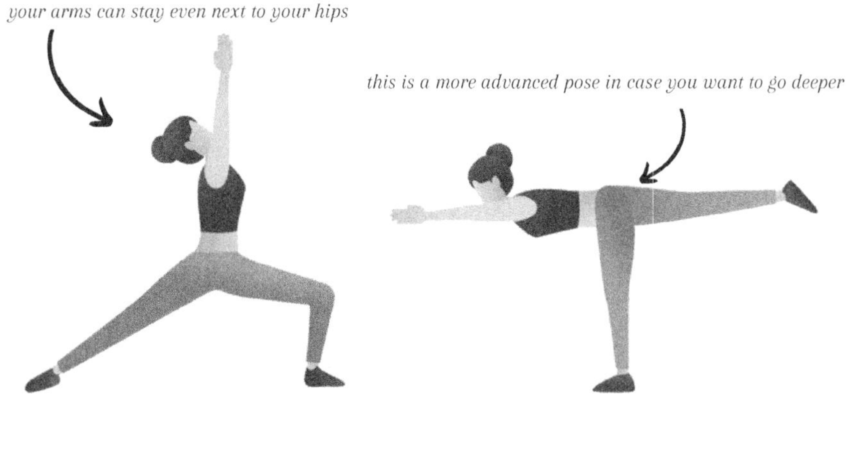

If you find yourself needing a visual reference for any of the exercises, a simple search on a video platform like YouTube, using the name of the pose, can offer you supplementary guidance. This way, you can ensure you're performing each movement correctly and safely.

Butterfly Stretch

How to Perform the Butterfly Stretch

1. Starting Position: Sit on the floor with your spine straight and tall. Bring the soles of your feet together in front of you, drawing your heels as close to your body as comfortable.
2. Knee Position: Allow your knees to fall out to the sides, feeling a stretch in your inner thighs. If your knees are high off the ground, that's okay – flexibility will improve over time.
3. Intensifying the Stretch: Gently press down on your thighs or knees with your elbows or hands for a deeper stretch, but be careful not to force them down.
4. Maintain the Position: Hold the stretch for 20-30 seconds, breathing deeply and steadily. Focus on relaxing your muscles with each exhale.
5. Avoid Bouncing: Keep the stretch static – avoid bouncing your knees up and down.
6. Exiting the Stretch: To release, slowly lift your knees, bring your legs together, and shake them out gently.

Butterfly Stretch

Tips

- Ensure that you're seated comfortably. You can sit on a cushion or folded blanket for added support.
- Keep your back straight throughout the stretch to prevent any strain on your spine.
- If you feel any pain or discomfort, ease off the stretch a bit. Stretching should involve a gentle pull, not pain.
- For an additional stretch, you can lean your torso forward from your hips while keeping your back straight. This motion deepens the stretch in your inner thighs and hips.
- As with any static stretch, focus on relaxing into the stretch rather than pushing too hard. Over time, your flexibility will naturally increase.

Note

The Butterfly Stretch is a fantastic static stretch for the inner thighs and hips. It's especially beneficial for those who require increased hip flexibility, such as runners, cyclists, or anyone who sits for long periods. Regular practice of this stretch can improve hip mobility, reduce tightness in the inner thighs, and promote overall lower body flexibility.

If you want a deeper stretch you can try this version

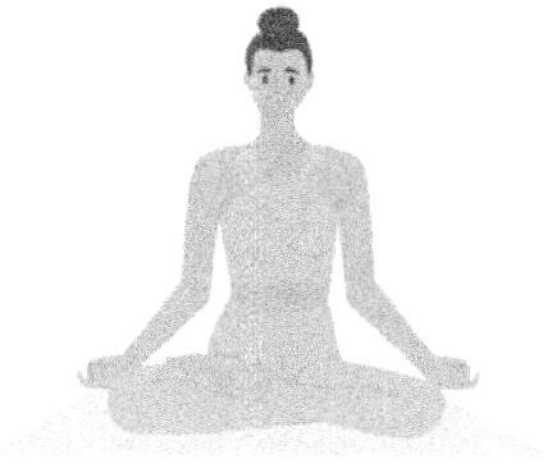

If you find yourself needing a visual reference for any of the exercises, a simple search on a video platform like YouTube, using the name of the pose, can offer you supplementary guidance. This way, you can ensure you're performing each movement correctly and safely.

Lunge with a Twist

How to Perform Lunge with a Twist

1. Starting Position: Stand with your feet together and your hands on your hips. Keep your back straight and your shoulders relaxed.
2. Step into a Lunge: Take a large step forward with your right foot, bending your knee to about a 90-degree angle. Your front thigh should be parallel to the floor, and your back leg should be straight with the heel lifted off the ground.
3. Perform the Twist: As you lunge, extend your arms out to the sides at shoulder height. Then, twist your upper body to the right, keeping your arms parallel to the floor. Turn your head to look over your right shoulder if it's comfortable.
4. Return to Starting Position: Untwist your upper body and bring your arms back to your sides. Push off your right foot to return to the starting position.
5. Repeat on the Other Side: Repeat the movement, this time stepping forward with your left foot and twisting to the left.
6. Rhythm and Breathing: Coordinate your movements with your breathing. Inhale as you step into the lunge and exhale as you twist.

Lunge with a Twist

Tips

- Keep your front knee aligned with your front ankle and ensure it doesn't extend past your toes to prevent strain.
- Engage your core muscles during the twist to support your spine and enhance the stretch.
- The twist should be gentle and controlled. Avoid over-rotating your torso.
- Keep your neck in a neutral position, in line with your spine, and avoid straining it as you turn your head.
- If balancing is challenging, perform the exercise near a wall or a chair for support.

Note

The Lunge with a Twist is an effective exercise for combining stretching and mobilization. It targets the leg muscles, hips, and spine, providing a dynamic stretch that enhances flexibility and encourages mobility in the torso. This exercise is particularly beneficial for loosening tight hip flexors and improving rotational movement in the upper body, making it a great addition to any warm-up or cool-down routine.

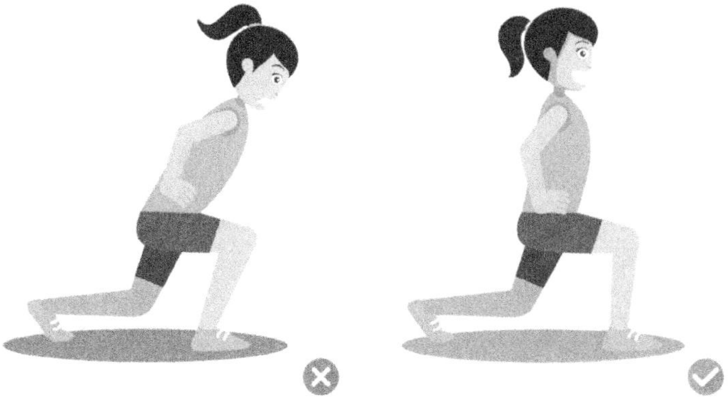

If you find yourself needing a visual reference for any of the exercises, a simple search on a video platform like YouTube, using the name of the pose, can offer you supplementary guidance. This way, you can ensure you're performing each movement correctly and safely.

BASIC EXERCISES

Pelvic Tilts

How to Perform Pelvic Tilts

1. Starting Position: Lie on your back on a flat surface (use a yoga mat for comfort). Bend your knees with your feet flat on the floor, hip-width apart. Keep your arms at your sides with palms facing down.
2. Neutral Spine: Start by establishing a neutral spine position. There should be a slight, natural curve in your lower back, and your spine should not be pressed into the floor.
3. Engage Your Core: Tighten your abdominal muscles, drawing your navel towards your spine. This engagement is crucial for the effectiveness of the exercise.
4. Tilt Your Pelvis: Exhale as you gently tilt your pelvis towards your ribcage. This movement will flatten your lower back against the floor. Avoid lifting your hips off the floor – the movement is small and controlled.
5. Return to Neutral: Inhale and slowly release the tilt, returning your pelvis to the neutral starting position.
6. Repetitions: Perform this movement for 10-15 repetitions, focusing on slow and controlled tilts.

Pelvic Tilts

Tips

- It's important to keep the rest of your body relaxed. The movement should be isolated to your pelvis and lower back.
- Keep your breath steady and synchronized with your movements – exhale during the tilt and inhale as you return to neutral.
- Don't rush the tilts. The effectiveness of pelvic tilts comes from the quality of the movement, not the quantity.
- As you get more comfortable with the exercise, you can hold the tilt for a few seconds before returning to the neutral position.

Note

Pelvic tilts are a fundamental exercise for strengthening the core and the lower back. They are particularly beneficial for improving lumbar spine stability, which can help alleviate lower back pain. This exercise is also a great starting point for building a stronger core, which is essential for overall body strength and injury prevention. Regular practice of pelvic tilts can lead to improved posture and a more supportive base for various physical activities.

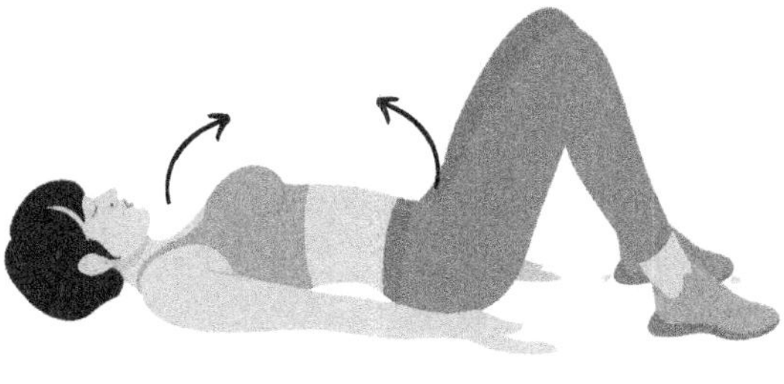

If you find yourself needing a visual reference for any of the exercises, a simple search on a video platform like YouTube, using the name of the pose, can offer you supplementary guidance. This way, you can ensure you're performing each movement correctly and safely.

Cat-Cow Stretch

How to Perform the Cat-Cow Stretch

1. Starting Position: Begin on your hands and knees in a tabletop position. Ensure your knees are set directly below your hips and your wrists, elbows, and shoulders are in line and perpendicular to the floor. Center your head in a neutral position, eyes looking at the floor.
2. Cow Pose: As you inhale, drop your belly towards the floor, lift your chin and chest, and gaze up toward the ceiling. In this position, you're making a concave shape with your spine.
3. Cat Pose: As you exhale, draw your belly to your spine and round your back toward the ceiling. The pose should look like a cat stretching its back. Release the crown of your head toward the floor, but don't force your chin to your chest.
4. Flowing Movement: Inhale, coming back into Cow Pose, and then exhale as you return to Cat Pose. Make the transition between these poses a smooth and fluid movement.
5. Rhythm and Breathing: Synchronize your movements with your breath, moving into Cow Pose on the inhale and into Cat Pose on the exhale. Continue for 1-2 minutes, following the natural rhythm of your breath.

Cat-Cow Stretch

Tips

- Keep your movements gentle and mindful. Do not rush the stretches or force your body into any positions that feel uncomfortable.
- Focus on the sensation of your spine arching and rounding. This exercise should feel good and help release tension in your back.
- Ensure that you keep your shoulders and knees in alignment to avoid any strain.
- If you have any neck issues, keep the head in line with the torso rather than dropping it back or forward.

Note

The Cat-Cow Stretch is excellent for enhancing spinal flexibility. It helps to gently stretch the spine, neck, and torso, while also massaging the organs in the belly. This exercise is a great way to start any workout routine as it warms up the body and brings increased awareness to the spine, a central area of movement in many exercises. Regular practice can lead to improved posture and relief from tension and stress in the back.

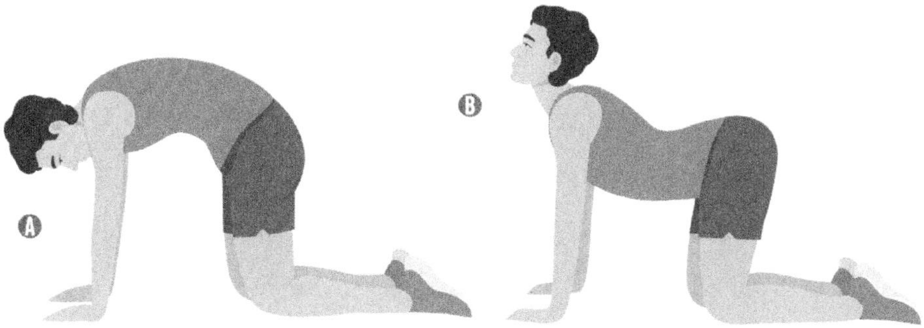

If you find yourself needing a visual reference for any of the exercises, a simple search on a video platform like YouTube, using the name of the pose, can offer you supplementary guidance. This way, you can ensure you're performing each movement correctly and safely.

Breath Awareness Exercise

How to Perform the Breath Awareness Exercise

1. Finding a Comfortable Position: Begin by finding a comfortable seated or lying down position. If seated, ensure your back is straight and your feet are flat on the floor. If lying down, lay flat on your back with your legs slightly apart and arms at your sides.
2. Relax Your Body: Close your eyes to help focus inward. Consciously relax your muscles, starting from your toes, moving up through your legs, torso, arms, and finally, your head.
3. Focus on Your Breathing: Place one hand on your chest and the other on your abdomen. This will help you focus on the movement of your diaphragm as you breathe.
4. Diaphragmatic Breathing: Inhale deeply through your nose, allowing your abdomen to rise as your lungs fill with air. Feel the hand on your abdomen rise, while the hand on your chest remains relatively still.
5. Exhale Slowly: Exhale slowly and completely through your mouth or nose, depending on what feels most comfortable. Feel the hand on your abdomen fall as you release the air.
6. Repeat: Continue to breathe deeply and slowly for several minutes. Focus your mind on the sensation of your breath entering and leaving your body, and the rise and fall of your abdomen.

Breath Awareness Exercise

Tips

- If your mind starts to wander, gently bring your focus back to your breathing. It's normal for the mind to drift, and the exercise includes returning your focus to your breath.
- Try to maintain a steady rhythm in your breathing, making your inhales and exhales of equal length.
- Diaphragmatic breathing not only aids in relaxation but also ensures efficient oxygen exchange and can improve respiratory and overall health.
- This exercise can be performed anytime you need to relax or refocus, such as before bed, upon waking up, or during breaks in your day.

Note

The Breath Awareness Exercise is centered on focusing on diaphragmatic breathing, which is a key component of stress reduction and relaxation. It encourages a deeper, more effective breathing pattern, which can have a calming effect on the nervous system. Regular practice can improve lung function, reduce stress levels, and enhance overall well-being. This exercise is also a foundational practice in many forms of meditation and yoga, emphasizing the connection between breath and mental clarity.

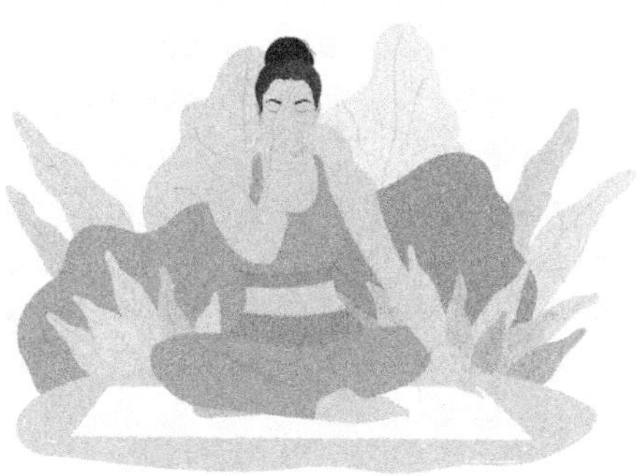

Knee-to-Chest Stretch

How to Perform Knee-to-Chest Stretch

1. Starting Position: Lie on your back on a flat, comfortable surface. Extend your legs straight out and relax your upper body, with your arms resting at your sides.
2. Bringing Knee to Chest: Bend your right knee and gently pull it towards your chest using both hands. Clasp your hands either behind your thigh or on top of your shin (but not on the knee cap) for support.
3. Hold the Stretch: Once you've brought your knee as close to your chest as comfortably possible, hold the position. You should feel a gentle stretch in your lower back and hip. Maintain this hold for about 20-30 seconds.
4. Return to Starting Position: Gently release your right leg and extend it back to the floor. Take a moment to relax before switching to the other leg.
5. Repeat with the Other Leg: Perform the same stretch with your left knee, following the same steps.
6. Alternate Legs: Continue to alternate between your right and left legs for a few repetitions.

Knee-to-Chest Stretch

Tips

- Ensure that your movements are slow and controlled. Avoid any sudden pulling or jerking motions.
- Keep your lower back pressed against the floor throughout the stretch to protect it and maximize the stretch on your hips.
- Breathe deeply and steadily as you perform this stretch. Deep breathing helps relax your muscles and deepens the stretch.
- If you experience any pain or discomfort, especially in the back or knee, ease off the stretch a bit.

Note

The Knee-to-Chest Stretch is a simple yet effective exercise for relaxing the lower back and hips. It helps alleviate tension and stiffness in these areas, which is especially beneficial for individuals who sit for long periods or have lower back discomfort. This stretch can also aid in improving hip flexibility and promoting overall relaxation in the lower body. Regular practice can contribute to a greater range of motion and comfort in daily movements.

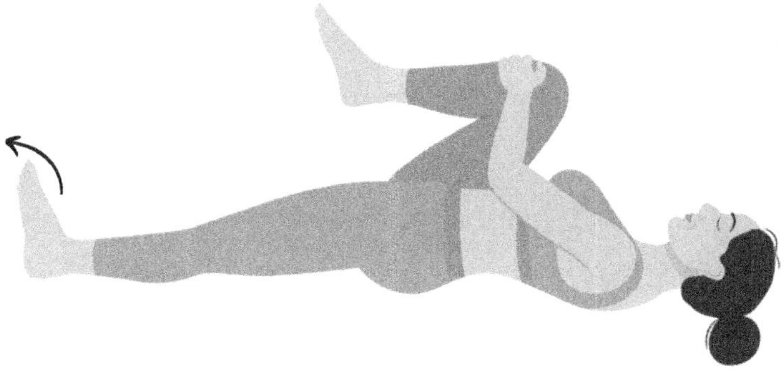

If you find yourself needing a visual reference for any of the exercises, a simple search on a video platform like YouTube, using the name of the pose, can offer you supplementary guidance. This way, you can ensure you're performing each movement correctly and safely.

Bridge Pose

How to Perform Bridge Pose

1. Starting Position: Lie on your back on a comfortable, flat surface. Bend your knees and place your feet flat on the ground, hip-width apart. Extend your arms along the floor with your palms facing down, your fingertips should be lightly touching your heels.
2. Lifting the Hips: Press your feet and arms firmly into the ground as you lift your hips towards the ceiling. Keep your thighs and feet parallel – resist the urge to let your knees splay outward.
3. Engage Your Muscles: As you lift your hips, engage your glutes and hamstrings. Be mindful to not overarch your lower back. Instead, focus on creating a straight line from your shoulders to your knees.
4. Upper Body Position: Keep your neck relaxed and your gaze upwards. Do not turn your head side-to-side while in the pose.
5. Hold the Pose: Hold Bridge Pose for 30 seconds to 1 minute. Breathe deeply and maintain a steady lift through your hips.
6. Lowering Down: To release the pose, slowly lower your hips back to the floor. Once down, hug your knees to your chest for a gentle counter-stretch.

Bridge Pose

Tips

- Ensure that your movements are smooth and controlled. Avoid jerky movements, especially when lifting into and lowering from the pose.
- If you feel any strain in your neck or back, reduce the height of your lift or place a folded blanket under your shoulders for support.
- To increase the intensity, clasp your hands under your back and press your arms down, lifting your hips higher.
- Keep your breath steady throughout the pose. This will help maintain a balance between effort and relaxation.

Note

Bridge Pose, or Setu Bandhasana, is an effective exercise for strengthening the back, glutes, and hamstrings. It also helps open up the chest and shoulders, which can be beneficial for those who spend a lot of time sitting. This pose can aid in improving posture and alleviating lower back pain. Regular practice of Bridge Pose can enhance core stability and contribute to a stronger, more balanced lower body.

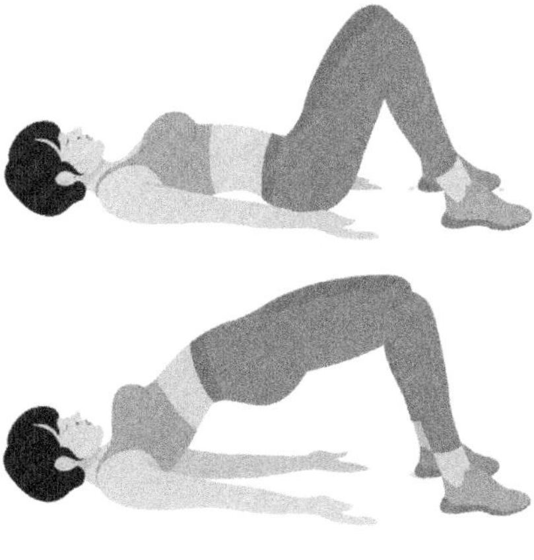

If you find yourself needing a visual reference for any of the exercises, a simple search on a video platform like YouTube, using the name of the pose, can offer you supplementary guidance. This way, you can ensure you're performing each movement correctly and safely.

INTERMEDIATE EXERCISES

Plank Pose

How to Perform Plank Pose

1. Starting Position: Begin in a tabletop position on your hands and knees. Place your wrists directly under your shoulders, and spread your fingers wide for a stable base.
2. Extend Your Legs: Step your feet back one at a time, extending your legs fully. Your body should form a straight line from your heels to the crown of your head.
3. Engage Your Core: Tighten your abdominal muscles to prevent your hips from sagging or lifting too high. Your body should be as straight as possible, resembling a plank.
4. Shoulder Position: Keep your shoulders engaged and away from your ears. Your neck should be in line with your spine, with your gaze down at the floor.
5. Hold the Pose: Maintain the plank position for 20-60 seconds, depending on your ability. Keep breathing steadily throughout the exercise.
6. To Release: To come out of the pose, either lower your knees to the floor or shift into a downward dog pose by lifting your hips up and back.

Plank Pose

Tips

- Ensure that your weight is evenly distributed between your hands and toes. Avoid putting too much pressure on your wrists.
- If holding a full plank is too challenging, modify by keeping your knees on the floor.
- Keep your legs active and your heels pressing back to maintain the integrity of the pose.
- To avoid straining your neck, keep your gaze fixed on a spot on the floor just in front of your hands.
- Practice regularly to gradually increase the duration of the pose.

Note

Plank Pose is a foundational exercise for building core and shoulder stability. It not only strengthens the abdominal muscles but also engages the shoulders, chest, legs, and back, making it an effective full-body exercise. Regular practice of Plank Pose can improve posture, enhance balance, and build endurance in the core muscles. This pose is also beneficial for supporting the spine and can be a key exercise for developing overall body strength and stability.

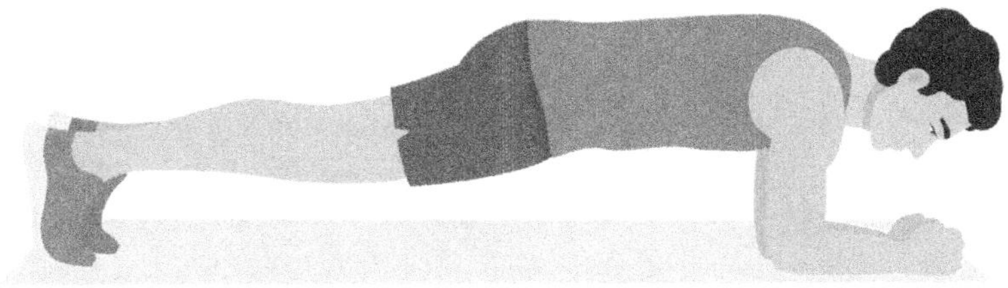

Leg Raises

How to Perform Leg Raises

1. Starting Position: Lie flat on your back on a comfortable, firm surface. Keep your legs extended and together. Place your arms at your sides with palms facing down for stability, or you can place your hands under your lower back for additional support.
2. Engage Your Core: Tighten your abdominal muscles to stabilize your spine. Press your lower back into the floor to avoid arching.
3. Raise Your Legs: Slowly lift your legs off the ground, keeping them straight. Raise them to a 90-degree angle with your body, or as high as you can without bending your knees or arching your back.
4. Lower Your Legs: Slowly lower your legs back to the starting position. Control the movement to avoid any jerking or dropping.
5. Breathing: Exhale as you lift your legs and inhale as you lower them back down. Keep your breath steady and controlled.
6. Repetitions: Start with a set of 10-15 leg raises. As your strength improves, you can increase the number of repetitions or sets.

Leg Raises

Tips

- Focus on the quality of the movement rather than the quantity. It's more effective to do fewer controlled leg raises than many quick, uncontrolled ones.
- Keep your movements slow and controlled to maximize the engagement of your abdominal muscles.
- If you feel any strain in your lower back, reduce the range of motion, or bend your knees slightly.
- Avoid lifting your hips off the floor as you raise your legs. The movement should come solely from your hip flexors and abdominal muscles.

Note

Leg raises are an effective exercise for strengthening the abdominal and hip muscles. They specifically target the lower abdominals, a region often challenging to engage with other exercises. Leg raises also help in improving hip flexibility and can contribute to a stronger, more stable core. Regular practice can enhance core endurance, which is beneficial for posture, balance, and overall athletic performance.

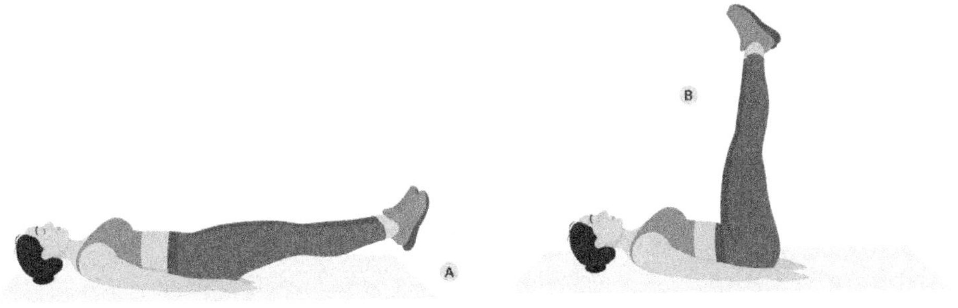

If you find yourself needing a visual reference for any of the exercises, a simple search on a video platform like YouTube, using the name of the pose, can offer you supplementary guidance. This way, you can ensure you're performing each movement correctly and safely.

Warrior II Pose

How to Perform Warrior II Pose

1. Starting Position: Begin standing with your feet together. Take a large step back with your right foot, keeping your left foot pointing forward. Your right foot should be turned outwards, approximately 90 degrees.
2. Aligning the Pose: Align your left heel with the arch of your right foot. Ensure your hips are open to the side, facing the same direction as your right foot.
3. Lowering into the Pose: Bend your left knee until it is directly over your left ankle, forming a right angle. Your right leg should remain straight.
4. Arm Position: Extend your arms out to the sides at shoulder height, keeping them parallel to the floor. Gaze over your left hand.
5. Holding the Pose: Hold this position, breathing deeply, for 30 seconds to 1 minute. Maintain a strong, grounded stance while keeping your upper body relaxed.
6. Return to Starting Position: To release the pose, straighten your left knee, lower your arms, and step your feet back together.
7. Repeat on the Other Side: Repeat the same process on the opposite side, stepping back with your left foot and bending your right knee.

Warrior II Pose

Tips

- Keep your front knee aligned with your front ankle to avoid straining the knee joint.
- Press down through the outer edge of your back foot for stability.
- Engage your core muscles to help maintain balance and support your upper body.
- Keep your shoulders relaxed and away from your ears, and your arms strong and active.
- If you feel unsteady, shorten your stance or perform the pose near a wall for support.

Note

Warrior II Pose, also known as Virabhadrasana II, is a powerful stance that builds lower body strength and balance. It targets the legs, hips, and ankles, while also stretching the chest and shoulders. This pose is excellent for improving stability and endurance, and it also encourages focus and concentration. Regular practice of Warrior II can enhance overall body alignment and posture.

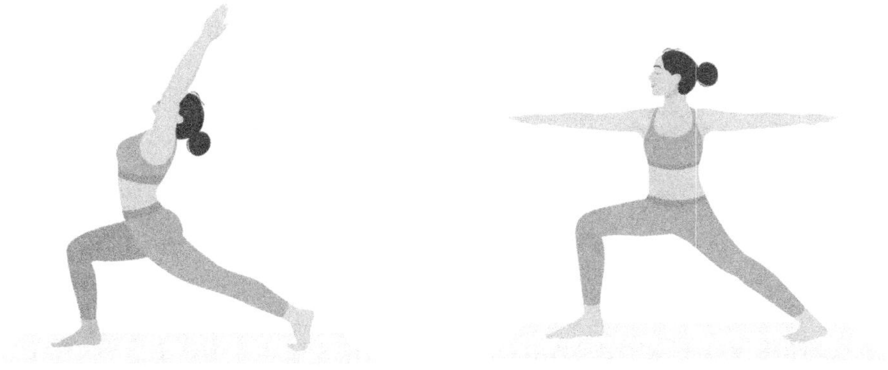

If you find yourself needing a visual reference for any of the exercises, a simple search on a video platform like YouTube, using the name of the pose, can offer you supplementary guidance. This way, you can ensure you're performing each movement correctly and safely.

Pigeon Pose

How to Perform Pigeon Pose

1. Starting Position: Begin in a tabletop position on your hands and knees.
2. Move into the Pose: Slide your right knee forward between your hands. Angle your right knee at two o'clock and place your right ankle near your left hip. Extend your left leg straight back behind you, keeping your hips square to the floor.
3. Adjust Your Position: If your right hip does not comfortably reach the floor, place a folded blanket or cushion underneath for support. This will help maintain alignment and prevent strain.
4. Upper Body Position: Initially, keep your torso upright and hands placed on the floor for balance. Inhale deeply as you lengthen your spine.
5. Forward Bend (Optional): For a deeper stretch, exhale and slowly walk your hands forward, bringing your torso down towards the floor. Rest your forehead on your hands or the floor, whichever is comfortable.
6. Hold the Pose: Stay in this position for 30 seconds to a minute, allowing your body to relax and sink deeper into the stretch with each exhale.
7. To Release: Gently walk your hands back, lifting your torso. Slide your right knee back to return to a tabletop position. Repeat the pose with your left knee forward.

Pigeon Pose

Tips

- Ensure that your back leg is aligned straight behind you and not angled to one side.
- Keep your front foot flexed to protect your knee joint.
- Breathing is key in Pigeon Pose. Deep, steady breaths will help you relax into the stretch.
- If you feel any sharp pain, especially in the knee, come out of the pose and consider a modified version or a different hip-opening exercise.
- Regularly practicing Pigeon Pose on both sides can help maintain balance in your hip flexibility.

Note

Pigeon Pose, or Eka Pada Rajakapotasana, is a deep stretching pose for the hips and glutes. It is highly beneficial for people who spend long periods sitting, as it effectively opens the hip flexors and rotators. The pose also stretches the thighs, groin, and psoas, and can relieve tension and tightness in the lower back. Regular practice of Pigeon Pose can enhance flexibility in the lower body, promote circulation, and contribute to overall hip health.

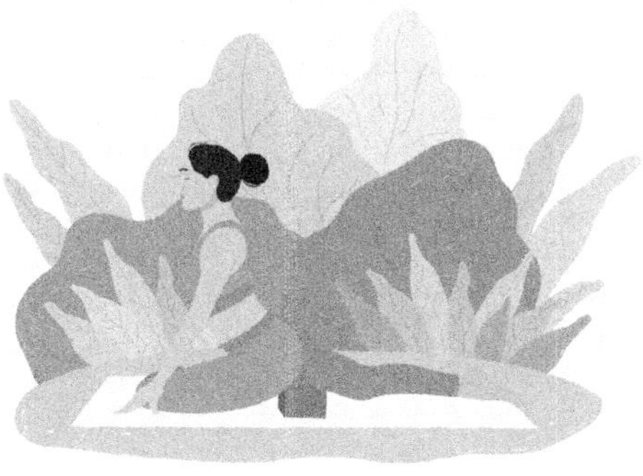

If you find yourself needing a visual reference for any of the exercises, a simple search on a video platform like YouTube, using the name of the pose, can offer you supplementary guidance. This way, you can ensure you're performing each movement correctly and safely.

Inverted Shoulder Stand

How to Perform Inverted Shoulder Stand

1. Starting Position: Begin by lying on your back on a comfortable surface. Place your arms at your sides, palms down for support.
2. Lift Your Legs: Bend your knees and bring them towards your chest. Gradually lift your hips off the floor, using your hands to support your lower back.
3. Straighten Your Body: Extend your legs upward, straightening your spine so that your body forms a straight line. Your weight should be supported by your shoulders, arms, and neck, not your head or neck.
4. Alignment: Keep your legs and spine as vertical as possible. Your chin should be tucked into your chest.
5. Hold the Pose: Maintain the pose for 30 seconds to a few minutes, depending on your comfort and experience level. Breathe deeply and steadily.
6. To Release: Gently lower your legs over your head into a plow pose, if possible, then slowly roll your spine back onto the floor, one vertebra at a time, using your hands for support.

Inverted Shoulder Stand

Tips

- Start with shorter durations and gradually increase as you become more comfortable with the pose.
- Keep the neck and head still throughout the pose to avoid strain. All the movement should come from the spine and hips.
- If you are a beginner, consider practicing near a wall or with the assistance of an experienced instructor.
- Avoid this pose if you have high blood pressure, neck issues, or are currently experiencing headaches or heart problems.

Note

Inverted Shoulder Stand, or Sarvangasana, is a powerful inversion known for its numerous benefits. It is particularly effective in improving circulation and balance. The pose encourages blood flow from the legs and pelvis back to the heart and then circulates it throughout the lungs and upper body, which can be revitalizing. Additionally, it strengthens the shoulders, back, and core muscles, enhancing overall stability and posture. Regular practice of Inverted Shoulder Stand can also help in calming the mind and relieving stress.

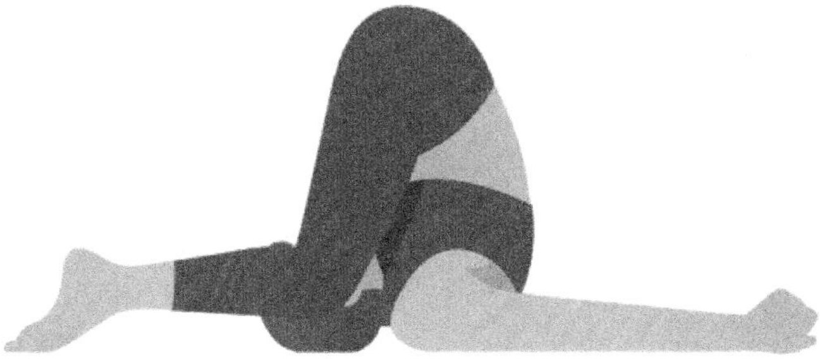

If you find yourself needing a visual reference for any of the exercises, a simple search on a video platform like YouTube, using the name of the pose, can offer you supplementary guidance. This way, you can ensure you're performing each movement correctly and safely.

4

INCORPORATING SOMATIC EXERCISES INTO DAILY LIFE

Incorporating somatic exercises into your daily life is a key step towards reaping their full benefits, particularly for beginners. Integrating these practices into your daily routine, both in the morning and evening can significantly enhance your overall well-being. The beauty of somatic exercises lies in their flexibility and adaptability, making them suitable for any time of the day. Morning routines in somatic exercises can be a refreshing way to start your day. These routines typically focus on gently waking up the body and mind, setting a positive tone for the day ahead. Morning practices include exercises that gently stretch and mobilize the body, helping to release any stiffness from sleep. Incorporating breathing techniques that energize the body, such as deep diaphragmatic breathing, can also be particularly effective in the morning. These routines don't have to be lengthy; even a few minutes of mindful movement can have a significant impact on your energy levels and mindset throughout the day. Evening routines, on the other hand, often focus on winding down and preparing the body for rest. Exercises for the evening might include more grounding and relaxing movements, helping to release the tension of the day. Practices that focus on slow, gentle stretches and calming breathing techniques can aid in relaxation and improve sleep quality. Evening routines can also be an excellent time for reflective practices, such as body scanning or mindfulness meditation, which encourage mental relaxation and a peaceful state of mind: the key to successfully incorporating somatic exercises into daily life is consistency and simplicity. Start with short, simple routines that are easy to remember and perform. As these practices become a regular part of your daily routine, you can gradually expand them, adding new exercises or extending the duration of your practice. It's also important to be flexible and listen to your body's needs. Some days, you might feel like doing a more energetic morning routine, while on other days, a gentle stretch might be all you need. Similarly, your evening routine might vary depending on how your body and mind feel at the end of the day.

Incorporating somatic exercises into your morning and evening routines is a way of honoring your body's needs and taking time for self-care. These practices not only improve physical health but also enhance mental clarity and emotional well-being. By making somatic exercises a regular part of your day, you embark on a continuous journey of self-discovery and holistic health.

Somatic exercises are efficient for stress relief and relaxation, making them an invaluable tool in our often hectic lives; understanding how to utilize these exercises specifically for calming the mind and body can be transformative. The gentle, mindful nature of somatic practices makes them ideal for releasing tension, both physical and mental. Stress, a common ailment in today's fast-paced world, manifests not just mentally but also physically. When we're stressed, our bodies tend to hold tension, often in the shoulders, neck, and back. Somatic exercises address this tension directly, using slow, deliberate movements that encourage the muscles to relax. By focusing on releasing this physical tension, we can also alleviate mental stress, as the body and mind are intricately connected. Breathing plays a critical role in using somatic exercises for stress relief. Deep, mindful breathing is a core element of these practices, helping to activate the body's natural relaxation response. Exercises that emphasize breath work, such as diaphragmatic breathing or paced breathing, can be efficient for calming the nervous system and reducing stress. Mindfulness, another essential aspect of somatic exercises, also contributes significantly to stress relief. By bringing your full attention to the present moment and the sensations in your body, you can break the cycle of chronic stress and anxiety. This mindful approach helps you step away from stressful thoughts and immerse yourself in the here and now, where calm and relaxation can be found.

For beginners, incorporating somatic exercises for stress relief into your daily routine can be simple yet effective. Even dedicating a few minutes each day to these practices can make a significant difference in your overall stress levels. You might choose specific exercises that you find remarkably calming or spend some time each day focusing on deep, mindful breathing. In addition to their immediate calming effects, regular practice of somatic exercises can lead to long-term improvements in stress management. Over time, you'll develop a deeper understanding of how your body responds to stress and how to release it effectively. This can lead to a more relaxed state of being in your daily life, improved sleep, and an overall sense of well-being.

Developing a consistent practice and forming lasting habits with somatic exercises, can be a fulfilling journey towards sustained well-being. Consistency is key in any form of exercise. Still, it becomes even more crucial when the focus is as much on the mind and internal awareness as it is on physical movement. Here are some tips to help you establish and maintain a regular practice of somatic exercises.

Start Small and Build Gradually: It's essential to begin with small, manageable goals. This could mean starting with just a few minutes of practice each day or a few exercises that you feel comfortable with. As you grow more accustomed to the routines, you can gradually increase the duration and complexity of your practice.

Remember, the aim is to integrate these exercises into your life without feeling overwhelmed.

Create a Routine: Try to incorporate your somatic exercise practice into your daily routine at a specific time. Whether it's a morning stretch to start your day or a series of relaxing movements before bed, having a set time each day helps establish a habit. Consistency in timing not only helps in forming a habit but also conditions your mind and body to be prepared and receptive to the practice.

Designate a Practice Space: Having a dedicated space for your somatic exercises can make your practice feel more special and intentional. It doesn't have to be a large area – just a quiet, comfortable spot where you won't be disturbed. This space can serve as a physical reminder and motivator for your daily practice.

Keep It Enjoyable: Ensure that your practice remains enjoyable and something you look forward to. Feel free to adjust the exercises to suit your mood and energy levels. Incorporating variety and allowing yourself the flexibility to adapt the practice can keep it interesting and engaging.

Track Your Progress: Keeping a journal or log of your practice can be motivational. Note down what you did, how long you practiced, and how you felt before and after. Over time, you'll be able to see the progress you've made, which can be incredibly encouraging.

Be Patient and Kind to Yourself: Remember that developing a new habit takes time. There will be days when you skip your practice or find it difficult to focus. It's important to be patient and not too hard on yourself during these times. Acknowledge that this is part of the process, and stay committed to your practice.

Use Reminders and Prompts: Setting reminders on your phone or leaving visual cues in places you frequent can be helpful. These reminders prompt you to take a few moments to practice, especially on busy days when somatic exercises might slip your mind.

Connect with a Community: Connecting with others who are on a similar journey can be motivating. Whether it's a local group or an online community, sharing experiences and tips can provide support and encouragement.

By incorporating these tips into your approach to somatic exercises, you can develop a consistent practice that becomes a natural and rewarding part of your daily life. Over time, this consistency in practice will not only enhance your physical well-being but also promote mental and emotional balance.

5

YOUR 28-DAY SOMATIC EXERCISE DIARY

Over the next 28 days, this diary is your space to choose the exercises that resonate with you the most, creating a practice that is uniquely yours.

Crafting Your Routine

Each day, you have the freedom to select exercises from the ones you've learned, focusing on those that bring you comfort and joy. There's no set routine to follow – instead, you listen to your body and choose movements that feel right for you on that particular day.

Your Daily Entries

For each day, write down the names of the exercises you choose to practice. Alongside, jot down the date and how you felt during and after the exercise. To make this process more intuitive and reflective, use the provided emoticons to express your feelings about the practice – whether it felt energizing, calming, challenging, or something else.

Flexibility and Adaptability in Practice

- Feel free to adjust the duration and intensity of each exercise to suit your energy levels and schedule.

- As you grow more comfortable, challenge yourself by exploring variations or progressing to more advanced movements.
- Always prioritize your comfort and safety, making adjustments or skipping exercises that don't feel right.

Consistency and Reflection

- Aim to incorporate somatic exercises into your daily life, even if it's just for a few minutes. Consistency is vital for experiencing the transformative effects of the practice.
- Use this diary to track your journey, noting not just the exercises but also the evolution of your feelings and experiences over the 28 days.

Revisiting and Repeating

Once you complete the 28-day cycle, feel free to revisit and repeat the exercises in any order. This diary is not just for a one-time journey; it's a tool for ongoing exploration and discovery.

Your journey with this diary is more than a physical fitness regimen; it's an opportunity to enhance your mind-body connection and embrace self-care. As you progress through these 28 days, you're not just improving your physical health; you're nurturing your mental well-being and enjoying a process that's centered around your personal growth and happiness.

Let's begin this 28-day journey towards a healthier, more balanced you!

YOUR 28-DAY SOMATIC EXERCISE DIARY

Your greatest strength lies in the commitment to your health.

Date   Feeling ☹ ☹ 😐 🙂 🙂

Exercise 1	
Exercise 2	
Exercise 3	
Exercise 4	
Exercise 5	

Flexibility in the body mirrors flexibility in life.

Date

Feeling ☹ 🙁 😐 🙂 😊

Exercise 1	
Exercise 2	
Exercise 3	
Exercise 4	
Exercise 5	

Your journey to wellness begins with a single step.

Date *Feeling*

Exercise 1	
Exercise 2	
Exercise 3	
Exercise 4	
Exercise 5	

Believe in the power of your own strength.

Date

Feeling ☹ 🙁 😐 🙂 😀

Exercise 1	
Exercise 2	
Exercise 3	
Exercise 4	
Exercise 5	

Transform your challenges into victories, one pose at a time.

Date

Feeling ☹ ☹ 😐 🙂 😀

Exercise 1	
Exercise 2	
Exercise 3	
Exercise 4	
Exercise 5	

Let mindfulness be your foundation for change.

Date

Feeling ☹ 🙁 😐 🙂 😀

Exercise 1	
Exercise 2	
Exercise 3	
Exercise 4	
Exercise 5	

Every moment of movement is a step towards a better you.

Date　　　　　　　　Feeling ☹ 🙁 😐 🙂 😀

Exercise 1	
Exercise 2	
Exercise 3	
Exercise 4	
Exercise 5	

Balance in the body brings harmony to the soul.

Date

Feeling

Exercise 1	
Exercise 2	
Exercise 3	
Exercise 4	
Exercise 5	

Challenge yourself to reach new heights of well-being.

Date

Feeling ☹ 🙁 😐 🙂 😀

Exercise 1	
Exercise 2	
Exercise 3	
Exercise 4	
Exercise 5	

Transform challenges into opportunities for growth.

Date Feeling ☹ 🙁 😐 🙂 😊

Exercise 1	
Exercise 2	
Exercise 3	
Exercise 4	
Exercise 5	

In harmony with your body, find peace for your mind.

Date

Feeling ☹ ☹ 😐 🙂 🙂

Exercise 1	
Exercise 2	
Exercise 3	
Exercise 4	
Exercise 5	

Let your breath be your guide to inner peace.

Date

Feeling

Exercise 1	
Exercise 2	
Exercise 3	
Exercise 4	
Exercise 5	

Your journey to wellness is a path of self-love and discovery.

Date

Feeling 😟 🙁 😐 🙂 😀

Exercise 1	
Exercise 2	
Exercise 3	
Exercise 4	
Exercise 5	

Find strength in stillness and calm in action.

Date

Feeling ☹ 🙁 😐 🙂 😀

Exercise 1	
Exercise 2	
Exercise 3	
Exercise 4	
Exercise 5	

Find joy in the journey, not just the destination.

Date

Feeling ☹ 🙁 😐 🙂 😀

Exercise 1	
Exercise 2	
Exercise 3	
Exercise 4	
Exercise 5	

Your potential is limitless when you listen to your body.

Date   Feeling

Exercise 1	
Exercise 2	
Exercise 3	
Exercise 4	
Exercise 5	

Today's efforts are tomorrow's rewards.

Date Feeling

Exercise 1	
Exercise 2	
Exercise 3	
Exercise 4	
Exercise 5	

Physical strength paves the way for mental resilience.

Date

Feeling

Exercise 1	
Exercise 2	
Exercise 3	
Exercise 4	
Exercise 5	

Each day is a chance to create a healthier you.

Date *Feeling* ☹ ☹ 😐 🙂 🙂

Exercise 1	
Exercise 2	
Exercise 3	
Exercise 4	
Exercise 5	

Embrace the journey of self-discovery through movement.

Date   Feeling ☹ 🙁 😐 🙂 😀

Exercise 1	
Exercise 2	
Exercise 3	
Exercise 4	
Exercise 5	

In every stretch, find a space for personal growth.

Date

Feeling

Exercise 1	
Exercise 2	
Exercise 3	
Exercise 4	
Exercise 5	

Let your fitness journey be a reflection of self-love.

Date

Feeling

Exercise 1	
Exercise 2	
Exercise 3	
Exercise 4	
Exercise 5	

In the balance of body and mind, find your true center.

Date Feeling ☹ 🙁 😐 🙂 😀

Exercise 1	
Exercise 2	
Exercise 3	
Exercise 4	
Exercise 5	

Empower yourself through the discipline of practice.

Date Feeling ☹ 🙁 😐 🙂 😀

Exercise 1	
Exercise 2	
Exercise 3	
Exercise 4	
Exercise 5	

Every exercise is a love letter to your body.

Date

Feeling

Exercise 1	
Exercise 2	
Exercise 3	
Exercise 4	
Exercise 5	

Your body is a temple: honor it with movement and care.

Date

Feeling ☹ 🙁 😐 🙂 😊

Exercise 1	
Exercise 2	
Exercise 3	
Exercise 4	
Exercise 5	

Embrace each day as a new opportunity to strengthen your body and mind.

Date   Feeling ☹ ☹ 😐 🙂 🙂

Exercise 1	
Exercise 2	
Exercise 3	
Exercise 4	
Exercise 5	

6

PROGRESSING IN SOMATIC EXERCISES

This Chapter delves into an essential aspect of your journey: recognizing and celebrating progress. As you progress in somatic exercises, it's essential to acknowledge the strides you've made, no matter how small they may seem. This recognition not only boosts your motivation but also reinforces the positive impact these practices have on your overall well-being. Progress in somatic exercises can be subtle and might not always be measured in conventional ways, such as increased reps or more weight lifted. Instead, it often manifests as improved body awareness, greater ease of movement, or a more profound sense of relaxation and well-being. For instance, you might notice that a particular posture that initially felt awkward is now more comfortable, or you may find yourself moving through your daily activities with greater ease and less tension. Another sign of progress is an enhanced mind-body connection. You may become more attuned to the needs of your body, responding intuitively to its signals of comfort and discomfort. This growing awareness is a significant achievement, reflecting a deepening understanding of the principles of somatic exercises. It's also worth celebrating the emotional and mental benefits you experience. Somatic exercises are designed to promote not just physical health but also mental and emotional well-being. You might find yourself feeling calmer, more grounded, or more resilient in the face of stress. These shifts in your emotional landscape are just as significant as the physical changes and deserve to be acknowledged. Celebrating progress doesn't always have to be about grand gestures. It can be as simple as taking a moment to reflect on how you feel after practice, noting any positive changes in a journal, or even sharing your achievements with a friend or a support group. These acts of recognition serve as powerful affirmations of your commitment to your practice and your well-being. In some cases, progress means recognizing when it's time to challenge yourself further. As you become more comfortable with the foundational exercises, you should explore more advanced movements or incorporate longer practice sessions. This willingness to step out of your comfort zone is a clear sign of progress. It should be approached with the same mindfulness and attentiveness that you've cultivated in your practice.

This chapter encourages you to be mindful of and celebrate your progress in somatic exercises. Whether it's through physical, emotional, or mental improvements, every step forward is a testament to your dedication and effort. By acknowledging and celebrating these achievements, you reinforce the positive impacts of somatic exercises and set the stage for continued growth and development in your practice. Advancing to more complex exercises in somatic practice is a journey that should be approached thoughtfully and mindfully, especially for beginners. Knowing when and how to progress is crucial to ensuring that your practice continues to be both safe and beneficial.

When to Advance

Advancement in somatic exercises is less about adhering to a strict timeline and more about listening to and understanding your body's readiness. Certain signs indicate you might be ready to take your practice to the next level:

1. *Comfort with Basic Movements:* If you find that the basic exercises have become quite comfortable and you're able to perform them with ease, it might be time to explore more challenging movements.

2. *Increased Body Awareness:* As your awareness of your body's signals and responses grows and you feel more in tune with its capabilities, this can be a sign that you're ready to progress.

3. *Desire for More Challenge:* If you're feeling that your current routine no longer stimulates or challenges you and you're craving more, it's likely a good time to consider advancing your practice.

How to Advance

Once you've determined that you're ready to progress, the next step is to approach this advancement carefully:

1. *Gradual Progression:* Rather than making a big leap to much more challenging exercises, it's safer and more effective to progress gradually. This could mean making small modifications to the exercises you're already doing or introducing one new, more complex movement at a time.

2. *Focus on Quality:* As you advance, maintain a strong focus on the quality of your movements. It's better to perform a more challenging exercise with good form for a shorter time than to do it improperly for longer.

3. *Maintain Mindfulness:* As exercises become more complex, it's crucial to stay mindful and connected with your body. Continue to pay close attention to how each new movement feels and adjust accordingly.

4. *Seek Guidance When Necessary:* If you need help with how to advance your practice safely, consider seeking advice from a somatic exercise instructor. Professional guidance can ensure that you

progress in a way that's appropriate for your individual needs and goals.

5. *Listen to Your Body:* Always listen to your body and respect its limits. If a new exercise causes discomfort or pain, take a step back and reassess whether it's suitable for you at this stage.

Remember, advancing in somatic exercises is not just a physical process but also a mental and emotional one. It involves continued learning, adaptation, and a deeper exploration of the connection between your mind and body. By approaching this progression with patience, mindfulness, and a willingness to listen to your body, you can ensure that your somatic exercise practice continues to grow and evolve in a way that supports your overall well-being. As you continue to explore and deepen your practice in somatic exercises, encountering challenges and experiencing plateaus is a natural part of the journey, especially for beginners. Understanding how to address these moments effectively is crucial for maintaining motivation and ensuring continued growth in your practice. Challenges in somatic exercises can take various forms. You might find specific movements particularly difficult, or you may need help to maintain a consistent routine. Emotional and mental blocks can also present challenges, especially as somatic exercises often bring a heightened awareness of one's internal state. These hurdles, while they may seem daunting, are opportunities for learning and self-discovery. When facing a challenge, the first step is to approach it with curiosity rather than frustration. Ask yourself what this challenge is teaching you. Is it highlighting an area of physical tension or weakness that needs attention? Or is it perhaps revealing a need for more mental focus or emotional release? Understanding the nature of the challenge can guide you in how to address it. Plateaus, or periods where progress seems to stall, are also common. In these phases, it might feel like you're not making any advancements, or you might lose some of the initial excitement you had when starting your practice. It's important to recognize that plateaus are a normal part of any learning process.

They are often periods of integration, where your body and mind are assimilating the new skills and knowledge you've gained. To move past a plateau, consider varying your routine. Introducing new exercises or modifying existing ones can provide fresh stimuli for both your body and mind, reigniting your interest and engagement. Sometimes, taking a short break from your routine and then returning to it can also offer a new perspective and renewed enthusiasm. Another effective strategy is to revisit your goals and motivations. Remind yourself why you started practicing somatic exercises in the first place. Realigning with your initial intentions can provide a boost of motivation and a clearer focus for your practice. Furthermore, it's beneficial to celebrate the progress you've already made. Reflecting on where you started and recognizing the improvements you've achieved can be incredibly motivating. It's a reminder that progress isn't always linear and that growth can happen in many different forms. Lastly, seeking support from a community or a coach can be invaluable in overcoming challenges and plateaus. Sharing your experiences, challenges, and successes with others can provide new insights, encouragement, and a sense of connection.

Addressing challenges and plateaus in your somatic exercise practice is about embracing them as part of your growth journey. By approaching them with patience, curiosity, and a willingness to adapt, you can continue to evolve and deepen your practice in meaningful ways.

7

THE ROLE OF NUTRITION AND HYDRATION IN SOMATIC EXERCISES

This chapter takes an insightful dive into an often-overlooked aspect of any physical practice: the role of nutrition and hydration. While the focus of somatic exercises is predominantly on movement and mindfulness, what you fuel your body with is equally critical. The interplay of nutrition, hydration, and physical activity is a dance of balance, where each element supports and enhances the others. Nutrition in the context of somatic exercises isn't about strict dieting or rigorous meal plans. Instead, it's about understanding and respecting your body's needs, providing it with the right kind of nourishment to support your somatic practice. Good nutrition complements physical activity by supplying the necessary energy and aiding in the recovery and rebuilding process. A diet rich in whole foods, including a variety of fruits, vegetables, whole grains, lean proteins, and healthy fats, ensures a well-rounded intake of essential nutrients. These foods not only provide the energy needed for your exercises but also contribute to overall health, improving muscle function, joint health, and even mental clarity. Hydration, too, plays a pivotal role. Somatic exercises, like any physical activity, require adequate hydration for optimal performance and recovery. Water is essential for almost every bodily function, including regulating body temperature, transporting nutrients, and lubricating joints. Proper hydration ensures that your body can perform these functions efficiently, which is particularly important during exercise. Additionally, staying well-hydrated can enhance your ability to concentrate and maintain focus during your somatic practices, making your sessions more effective and enjoyable; incorporating good nutrition and hydration habits can be a gradual process. It's about making mindful choices, listening to your body, and responding to its needs. This might mean adjusting your water intake based on how active you are or noticing how different foods affect your energy levels and mood. The goal is to develop a relationship with food and water that supports and nourishes your body, complementing your somatic exercise practice. Moreover, the mindfulness cultivated through somatic exercises can be extended to eating and drinking habits. Just as somatic exercises encourage you to be present and aware of your body's movements, you can apply the same principles to eating and drinking. Paying attention to the tastes, textures, and sensations of eating not only enhances the experience but can also lead to more intuitive and healthful eating patterns. Nutrition and hydration are not just supplementary to your somatic exercises; they are integral components of a holistic approach to wellness. By nourishing your body with the right foods and ensuring adequate hydration, you provide a strong foundation for your somatic practice. This chapter aims to guide you in understanding and integrating these essential aspects into your daily routine, enhancing both your somatic exercises and your overall well-being. Sleep, often underestimated in its importance, is a powerful tool for wellness. It's during sleep that the body undergoes repair and rejuvenation. Muscles that have been exercised and stretched during somatic practices heal and strengthen during rest periods. Moreover, sleep plays a vital role in cognitive functions, including memory consolidation and emotional processing. Good quality sleep enhances your ability to learn and retain the new skills you acquire in your somatic exercise practice.

Establishing a healthy sleep routine can significantly enhance the effectiveness of somatic exercises. It's not just the quantity of sleep that matters, but also its quality. Practices from your somatic exercise routines, especially those focused on relaxation and stress reduction, can be highly beneficial in improving sleep quality. Exercises that promote relaxation can be incorporated into your evening routine to help transition your body into a state conducive to restful sleep. Recovery, too, is an essential aspect of any physical practice, including somatic exercises. While somatic practices are generally gentle and low impact, giving your body time to rest and recover is crucial. This doesn't necessarily mean complete rest or inactivity but involves engaging in activities that are vital rather than strenuous. It can include practices like gentle stretching, mindful walking, or even relaxation techniques. In somatic exercises, understanding the signs of your body needing rest and recovery is key. This might include feelings of tiredness, soreness, or a general lack of energy. Respecting these signals and allowing your body the time it needs to recover not only prevents injuries but also makes your practice more sustainable and enjoyable in the long run; recovery is not just physical. Somatic exercises, with their emphasis on the mind-body connection, underscore the importance of mental and emotional recovery as well. Engaging in activities that you find relaxing and enjoyable, such as reading, meditating, or spending time in nature, can be highly beneficial. These activities can help clear your mind, reduce stress, and enhance your overall well-being.

Sleep, and recovery are not merely adjuncts to your somatic exercise practice; they are integral to it. They form the foundation upon which the benefits of the exercises are built. By prioritizing sleep and recovery, you ensure that your body and mind are adequately rested and prepared for the demands of somatic exercises. This chapter aims to provide insights and guidance on integrating these crucial aspects into your wellness routine, enhancing both your somatic practice and your overall quality of life. The connection between somatic practices and emotional health is a profound and integral aspect of the journey into somatic exercises, especially for beginners.

Somatic practices go beyond physical wellness, delving into the realms of emotional and mental well-being. This holistic approach recognizes that our emotional state is deeply intertwined with our physical state, and by addressing one, we can significantly impact the other. Somatic exercises, with their emphasis on mindfulness and body awareness, offer a unique pathway to emotional health. These practices encourage you to tune into your body's sensations and responses, fostering a deep sense of connection with yourself. This reflective process often leads to greater emotional awareness. You become more attuned to how emotions manifest in your body – perhaps as tension in specific muscles, changes in breathing patterns, or overall energy levels. By becoming aware of these physical manifestations of emotions, you can begin to understand and process your feelings more effectively. Somatic practices provide a safe and gentle way to release stored emotions. It's not uncommon for individuals to hold emotional tension in their bodies, sometimes without even realizing it. Through mindful movement and focused breathing, somatic exercises can help release this tension, offering a sense of relief and emotional release. This process can be particularly empowering for those who may find it challenging to express emotions verbally; the emotional benefits of somatic exercises can be incredibly impactful. As you start to practice, you might notice shifts in your emotional landscape – perhaps a sense of calm after a session, a release of pent-up stress, or a newfound sense of emotional balance. These changes are as significant as any physical improvement. They are a vital part of the transformative power of somatic exercises. The practices also foster resilience and emotional regulation. By regularly engaging in somatic exercises, you develop tools to manage stress, anxiety, and other emotional challenges more effectively. The skills you learn – such as mindful breathing, body scanning, and movement with awareness – can be applied in everyday life, helping you navigate emotional ups and downs with greater ease.

The connection between somatic practices and emotional health is a key component of the holistic approach these exercises embody. This chapter not only highlights the physical aspects of somatic exercises but also delves into how these practices can support and enhance emotional well-being. By embracing this connection, you can embark on a journey that nourishes your body, calms your mind, and uplifts your spirit.

AFTERWORD

As we reach the end of "Somatic Exercises for Beginners," it's a time for reflection, not just on the exercises and techniques learned, but on the broader journey you've embarked upon. This journey into somatic practice is about much more than physical movements; it's about cultivating a deeper connection with yourself, embracing lifelong learning, and continuing to explore and grow in your practice. Reflecting on your journey thus far, you may notice the subtle yet profound ways in which somatic exercises have begun to influence your life. You may find yourself moving with greater ease, experiencing less tension, or feeling more present and mindful in your daily activities. These changes, whether big or small, are significant milestones in your journey. They signify a growing awareness and understanding of your body and how it interacts with your mind and emotions. Somatic exercises are not a static practice but a field rich with opportunities for lifelong learning. As you continue your journey, you'll find that there is always more to discover and explore. Each movement, each breath, and each moment of mindfulness offers a chance to deepen your understanding and refine your practice. This ongoing learning process is one of the most rewarding aspects of somatic exercises, as it continually opens new doors to personal growth and well-being.

Your journey doesn't end with this book. Instead, it marks the beginning of a lifelong exploration into somatic practices. There are always new levels of awareness to reach, new movements to master, and deeper insights into the mind-body connection to uncover. The field of somatic exercises is vast and varied, offering a rich tapestry of practices to explore. Whether it's delving deeper into the techniques you've already learned or branching out into other somatic disciplines, there is a wealth of knowledge and experience waiting for you. As you move forward, remember that the practice of somatic exercises is a personal journey, one that is unique to you. Listen to your body, trust your intuition, and allow your practice to evolve in a way that best supports your needs and goals. Be open to trying new things, but also be patient with yourself. The beauty of somatic exercises lies in their gentle approach, which respects and honors the body's wisdom and timeline. I encourage you to maintain your practice and exploration of somatic exercises. Keep making space for it in your life, as it is a valuable tool for maintaining physical, mental, and emotional health. Your journey in somatic practice is one of continual discovery, offering endless opportunities for growth, healing, and joy.

Thank you for allowing "Somatic Exercises for Beginners" to be a part of your journey. May you continue to find fulfillment, balance, and well-being in your ongoing exploration of somatic practices.

If you found this book helpful, please leave a review on Amazon. Your feedback is not only greatly appreciated, but it also helps others discover this resource and embark on their paths to health and wellness. Sharing your experience and the impact this book has had on your journey can be incredibly inspiring and motivating to others looking to make similar changes in their lives.

Thank you once again for choosing this book as a companion on your wellness journey. Here's to your continued health and happiness!

Printed in Great Britain
by Amazon

37052208R00076